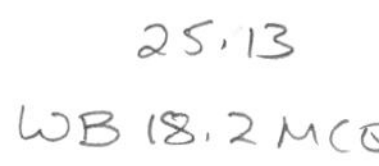

QNOTES FOR THE MRCP PART 1

QNOTES FOR THE MRCP PART 1

by

Raymond McCrudden BSc(Hons) MRCP

Editor and Author
Registrar in Gastroenterology
St Vincent's Hospital
Sydney
NSW Australia

With contributions from

John Gordon MRCP

Research Fellow in Immunology
Southampton University Hospitals Trust
Southampton

Callum Pearce MRCPI

Research Fellow in Gastroenterology
Queen Alexandra Hospital
Portsmouth

Lynn Thomas BSc(Hons) MRCP

Registrar in Rheumatology and General Medicine
Queen Alexandra Hospital
Portsmouth

QNOTES FOR THE MRCP
PART 1

QBase series developed and edited by

Edward J Hammond MA BM BCh MRCP FRCA

Department of Anaesthetics
Royal Devon & Exeter NHS Trust

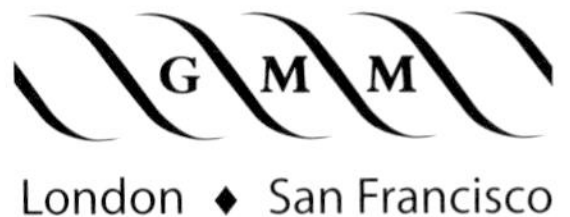

London ♦ San Francisco

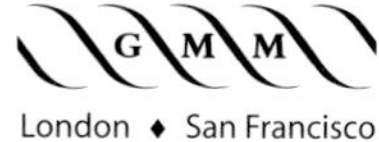

Greenwich Medical Media Ltd.
137 Euston Road
London
NW1 2AA

ISBN 184110 0994

First Published 2002

A catalogue record for this book is available from the British Library

Produced and Designed by
Saxon Graphics Limited, Derby

Printed in the UK by
Ashford Colour Press Ltd

www.greenwich-medical.co.uk

Distributed worldwide by Plymbridge Distributors Ltd
and in the USA by JAMCO Distribution

Contents

QNotes MRCP Part 1

QNotes MRCP Part 1 has been designed as a companion volume to the Royal College of Physicians MRCP (UK) Part 1 Papers 1997/98 CD-ROM.

QNotes is based on the QBase Interactive MCQ Examinations program and retains all of its functions. Before installing QNotes you must install the QBase MRCP Part 1 Papers 1997/98 CD-ROM onto your computer. Q Notes MRCP Part 1 should only be used with the QBase MRCP Part 1 Papers CD in the CD-ROM drive of your computer. QNotes runs from your hard disk, reads the exam papers and questions from the Part 1 Papers CD-ROM and attaches comprehensive notes to each question.

Installation Instructions

Before using QNotes MRCP Part 1 you must install the Royal College Physicians MRCP Part 1 Papers 1997/98 onto your computer

Put the MRCP Part 1 Papers CD in the CD drive of your computer and double click the setup.exe to run the QBase installer.

Remove the MRCP Part 1 Papers CD and insert the QNotes MRCP Part 1 CD into the CD drive.

View the contents of the QNotes CD-ROM.

Copy the folder labelled QNotes MRCP Part 1 onto your desktop (*do not change the names of any of the files or folders within this folder*).

Remove the QNotes CD from the CD drive and replace it with the MRCP Part 1 Papers CD.

You can now run QNotes from your hard disk by double clicking the QNotes program file.

Q Notes will enhance the value of the questions contained on the Part 1 Papers CD by seamlessly attaching comprehensive notes to them.

*See **Readme.txt** in the QNotes MRCP Part 1 folder for further information.*

The Royal College of Physicians is removing negative marking from May 2002, but the format of the MRCP Part 1 examination will remain the same. A non-negatively marked version of *QNotes* will be available shortly on *www.greenwich-medical.co.uk/qnotes.*

Editor's Note

Before you use QNotes, please follow the installation instructions carefully.

QNotes has been designed to add comprehensive and updateable notes to QBase publications. QNotes has been developed as an extension to the QBase Interactive MCQ Examinations program designed to facilitate revision for postgraduate medical exams. QBase was used by the Royal College of Physicians to release its Part 1 Papers in 2000 on CD-ROM.

QNotes MRCP Part 1 has been designed specifically as a companion volume to the Royal College of Physicians MRCP Part 1 Papers Book/CD. QNotes MRCP Part 1 seamlessly integrates comprehensive notes and explanations with the questions contained on the MRCP Part 1 Papers CD. In order for QNotes MRCP Part 1 to work you must have the Royal College of Physicians MRCP Part 1 Papers 97/98 CD in your CD drive.

The QNotes program will run from your hard disk. QNotes contains all the same functions as QBase. Previous users of QBase will be familiar with the ability to choose predefined exams, set their own mock exams or select questions from a choice of subjects. QNotes will integrate the appropriate notes and explanations with all the questions on the MRCP Part 1 Papers CD and enhance your learning experience. If you have not used QBase before please refer to the Helpfile contained on either the Part 1 Papers or the QNotes CD or press the appropriate button on the quick start menu.

The QNotes/QBase series of books and CDs have been designed to facilitate your revision and learning experience. Unlike traditional book publications the Interactive MCQ Program gives candidates the option and flexibility to make up their own exam papers for revision or assessment. Questions can be selected from the entire pool based on the user's choice of subject and format rather than the fixed order of traditional book publishing. Although the exam format and marking system continue to evolve, the core subject matter under examination remains much the same. QBase and QNotes will continue to evolve in parallel with changes in the format and marking systems of the different Royal Colleges.

We continue to value the views of candidates, past and present on how we can improve the program. If you have any suggestions, comments or technical problems with QBase please contact us via email at gm@greenwich-medical.co.uk.

We hope that candidates will find that QNotes will facilitate their revision for the MRCP Part 1 examination.

Good Luck!

Edward Hammond and Ray McCrudden
February 2002

Acknowledgments

I would like to thank my co-authors, John, Callum and Lynn who each contributed an equal 25% share to the workload. This book has taken a slightly longer time to write than anticipated, but for good reason. By the time this is published three out of the four of us will have embarked on the journey taken by all who start a young family: I for one can identify now with those tired parents who come to work looking exhausted and complaining of little sleep. And I for one wouldn't have it any other way. I want to thank my co-authors for their work during times when they would rather have caught up with rest in a horizontal frame of mind or spent some well-earned time with their partner and children.

Thanks also to Ed Hammond for dragging another book out of me and also to Gavin Smith and Gill Clark at Greenwich Medical who were *very* patient with the multiple delays and deadlines revisited etc. A special thanks to John Iredale, David Fine and Michael Arthur in Southampton and David Williams and Miriam Levy in Sydney for inspiration and support.

A big thank you to Herman and Anne at 'The Mill' for putting up with me whilst writing during an Autumn sojourn in Stuttgart, and to my parents Raymond and Audrey for their help despite the long distance from the UK who have supported us during our work here in Sydney and in the writing of this book. Finally the biggest Thank You goes to my wife Ute and son Nicolas who put up with multiple weekends writing: the ultimatum was to finish before the 'next one' – I think we have succeeded … just.

RM
Sydney
March 2002

Preface

This book has been written with the sole aim of annotating the questions, published by Greenwich Medical Media, of the Royal College of Physicians (UK) exam, Membership of the Royal College Part I (MRCP I), for the years 1997 and 1998. In addition to detailed notes on any given topic, each question is referenced, directing the reader to up to date reviews or papers on the subject should they wish to research the area further. In addition to the book a CD-ROM is provided which, once installed to the hard drive on your computer, complements the CD-ROM provided in the College Questions published by Greenwich Medical Media last year (you will still need the original College CD-ROM containing the college questions).

Recently the exam format of the MRCP I has altered and whilst the current QBase program still has the facility to help candidates examine and improve their technique in guessing, by far the greatest advantage of the program is to allow the candidate to do an exam paper 'on screen', choose the format of the exam, store the paper for later use, and finally to identify from the answers areas of weakness that require attention.

Medicine and the Internet

One of the themes put forward in QBase Medicine II was the use of computers in medicine. In this preface the theme is developed further with the use of the internet as a resource for studying for the exam. There is no doubt that doing lots of multiple choice questions with focussed answers is the best preparation for the exam however very occasionally further information is required. In addition to textbooks and journals in the library the internet, if used wisely, can be a valuable resource. For those who are complete novices to the subject we have put together a document which serves as an introduction to gaining access to a variety of medical web sites on the internet (Appendix: Membership and the web). This text is also provided on the CD-ROM as a Microsoft Word file and also as a rich text file for those with other word processing applications: if it is installed onto a computer equipped for the internet, then by simply clicking on the 'hyperlink' text you will be taken to the web site in question.

Request for comments

Please give us feedback on the book whether it be typos, errors, misleading statements or additions to existing lists. This will help us in future editions.

You can send any 'bug reports' or comments to:

QNotes
(Annotations to the MRCP Part I College Questions published 1997, 1998)
Greenwich Medical Media Ltd
137 Euston Road
London
NW1 2AA

email to:
gm@greenwich-medical.co.uk

We hope that the time and effort taken in putting these answers together will impart a clarity and ease of understanding to the text, and help towards the final goal. Good luck!

Ray McCrudden
Callum Pearce
John Gordon
Lynn Thomas

March 2002

Paper 1 Answers

Question 1

A. false **B.** true **C.** true **D.** false **E.** false

Studies in molecular genetics have shown that mutations or deletions underlie some diseases such as:

1. Some forms of Alzheimers (point mutation in the gene for the amyloid precursor protein)
2. The spongiform encephalopathies such as Creutzfeldt-Jakob disease (mutations in the prion protein gene)
3. Familial amyotrophic lateral sclerosis (abnormalities in the superoxide dismutase gene)
4. Charcot Marie Tooth disease (reduplication of the chromosome 17 gene)
5. Duchenne and Becker muscular dystrophies (deletion of the dystrophin gene)
6. Mitochondrial DNA deletions underlie Lebers optic atrophy, Leighs necrotizing encephalopathy of childhood, and the mitochondrial myopathies.
7. Abnormal amplification of particular trinucleotide repeats occurs in X linked bulbospinal muscular atrophy, fragile X syndrome, myotonic dystrophy, Huntington's Chorea, Spinocerebellar ataxia type I, and Dentatorubral pallidoluysian atrophy. They share a progressive lengthening of the trinucleotide repeat (CGG, CAG, CTG) sequence from one generation to the next and at some critical length the associated gene malfunctions.

Syndrome	***Linkage***	***Anticipation***
Fragile X	X linked	Yes
Spinobulbar muscular atrophy	X linked	No
Myotonic dystrophy	Aut Dom	Yes
Huntingdons disease	Aut Dom	Yes
Spinocerebellar ataxia type I	Aut Dom	Yes
Fragile X	X linked	No
Dentatorubral pallidoluysian atrophy	Aut Dom	Yes

Myotonic dystrophy is a good example of a disease demonstrating anticipation in which there is increased severity at an earlier age of onset with successive generations. For example the grandparent may just have cataracts and the diagnosis will not be considered until the offspring presents with classical myotonia in early adult life. (In some cases it is difficult to decide which grandparent is affected). The grandchild however may have congenital disease (especially if the transmitting parent is the mother). A correlation exists between the age of onset and the length of the CTG repeat in the untranslated 3' end of the myotonin protein kinase gene.

Causes of optic atrophy

Hereditary	Lebers optic atrophy Dominant optic atrophy Retinitis pigmentosa Tay Sachs disease
Acquired	Trauma to optic nerve (e.g. birth hypoxia) Infections (meningitis, encephalopathies, neuropathies) Demylination disorders Pituitary tumours Meningiomas Toxins (methanol, quinine, tobacco amblyopia)

Pembrey ME. Genetic factors in disease
Oxford Textbook of Medicine. Oxford University Press

Question 2

A. false **B.** true **C.** false **D.** true **E.** true

Causes and associations of diabetes mellitus:

Primary causes:

Type I	insulin dependent
II	non insulin dependent
III	(limited to the tropics) malnutrition related

Secondary

pancreatitis (acute/chronic)
haemochromatosis
endocrine disorders producing excess levels of:
- cortisol (Cushing's syndrome)
- growth hormone (acromegaly)
- glucagon (glucagonoma)
- adrenaline (phaeochromocytoma)

Drug induced, certain genetic syndromes

Type I diabetes (IDDM), once termed juvenile type onset diabetes, is the result of an autoimmune destruction of the islets of Langerhans. It typically presents before 30 years, but it can occur at any age. It results in a very substantial destruction of the total capacity of the islet beta cells to secrete insulin. Islet cell antibodies are usually found in the plasma for a period of 1–2 years after diagnosis, but in a minority (20%) these may persist for the remainder of the patients life. Members of this subgroup, sometimes called type Ib, are particularly liable to suffer other autoimmune diseases e.g. coeliac disease or rheumatoid arthritis. In Ib there is a higher percentage of females and older age of onset. There is an association with HLA types e.g. DR3 (males) DR4 (females). Patients are mostly young and often markedly thin at diagnosis. In the early phase they retain some endogenous insulin secretion and may have a honeymoon phase; later there is no endogenous insulin. Ketoacidosis develops when insulin is withdrawn or during stress states.

Individuals at risk of developing IDDM can be identified by the presence of autoimmune serological markers, including islets cell antibodies, antibodies to insulin and glutamic acid decarboxylase (GAD) and a decline in beta cell insulin secretory capacity. GAD is an enzyme involved in the conversion of glutamate to γ-amino butyric acid, a key neuroendocrine transmitter. Antibodies to GAD are highly predictive of future IDDM and insulin dependency.

50% of all cases are diagnosed before 20 years of age. In adults the onset may be much slower and the disorder may mimic NIDDM. The risk that IDDM will develop before the age of 20 years is about 6% for a sibling of a patient with IDDM and 5% for a child whose father has IDDM. The risk for the child of a mother with IDDM is 2–3% (if she was diagnosed after the age of 8) but up to 22% if she was diagnosed before 8. The major locus is in the short arm of chromosome 6. 90% of Caucasians with IDDM have DR3 or DR4; DR2 is protective. HLA-DQ alleles are even more closely associated with IDDM:

HLA DR4-DQA*0301 DQB1*0302 and

HLA DR4 DQA1*0102 DQB1*0201 predispose to IDDM.

There is relative concordance in monozygotic twins in contrast to Type II diabetics where there is a strong concordance with identical twins in studies (>90%). IgM antibodies against coxsackie virus have been found in 25–30% of new cases, suggesting recent infection. Coxsackie virus B RNA has been detected in 65% of children under the age of 7 years with newly diagnosed IDDM, compared with 4% of controls, consistent with recent or persistent infection. Cytomegalovirus DNA sequences are incorporated into the genome in 22% of newly diagnosed diabetes, compared with 26% of controls.

Bell JI, Hockday TDR. Diabetes Mellitus
Oxford Textbook of Medicine. Oxford University Press.

Question 3

A. true **B.** true **C.** true **D.** false **E.** true

As suggested from the stem there is a missing chromosome in Turner's syndrome.

The incidence is around 1 in 2500–3500 of female births and presents either at birth or infancy or in mid childhood. Turner's syndrome is probably the most common chromosomal cause of osteoporosis and the commonest cause of ovarian dysgenesis.

Recognized features of Turner's syndrome:
Slight reduction in expected IQ range but great majority in the normal range
Osteoporosis
Hirsutism
Primary ovarian failure
Pubertal delay
Renal anomalies
Eye findings: epicanthus/ptosis
Short stature
Webbed neck
Shield chest with wide spaced nipples
Wide carrying angle of the arms
Congenital heart defect (esp. coarctation)
Café au lait spots
Black freckles/low hairline
Double layered eye lashes
Characteristically they have XO karyotype with reduced numbers of Barr bodies in the buccal smears
Hearing loss

It is now possible to provide women with Turner's syndrome with fertility through ovum donation, although the shortage of oocytes remains an important and usually critically limiting factor. Treatment for short stature involves a slow introduction of ethinyl oestradiol at the age of 12 to 13 for 2 years (omitting the dose 1 week in every 4 once adult doses are reached) with progesterone in the final week. For the lack of puberty recombinant human growth hormone and the mild anabolic steroid oxandrolone have been of benefit.

Causes of Primary ovarian failure:

Idiopathic
Turner's
Autoimmune disease (hypothyroidism, Addison's disease, IDDM)
Anticancer therapy
Resistant ovaries
Surgery
Radiotherapy
Galactosaemia
Familial
Miscellaneous

Causes of short stature:

Proportionate	
Genetic	familial
Endocrine	lack of growth hormone, hypothyroidism
Metabolic	lysosomal storage diseases
	renal glomerular failure, cystic fibrosis
Nutritional	coeliac disease, starvation
Chronic disease	cyanotic heart disease
Intrauterine	low birth weight dwarfism
Chromosomal	Turner's
Social	emotional deprivation

Disproportionate	
Short limbs	
Lethal	type II osteogenesis imperfecta
	thanatophoric dwarfism
	achondrogenesis
Non-lethal	achondroplasia
	inherited hypophosphataemia
	metaphyseal dystosis
Short spine	spondyloepiphyseal dysplasia

Preece MA. Normal growth and its disorders
Oxford Textbook of Medicine. Oxford University Press.

Question 4

A. true **B.** true **C.** false **D.** false **E.** false

Down's syndrome is characterised by an extra chromosome where the karyotype is written 47,XX+21, or 47,XY+21 if male. 96% are due to primary non-dysjunction, 95% of these involve errors in the formation of the ovum rather that the sperm. Down's syndrome has an incidence of 1 in 1,200 mothers less than 30 years to about 1 in 100 at the age of 39 years. If a couple have 1 child with Down's there is a 1 in 100 chance of another trisomy, usually Down's. Other examples of trisomies include: Trisomy 18 (Edwards syndrome) and trisomy 13 (Patau syndrome).

In 2–3% of cases there is a chromosome translocation (usually a Robertsonian translocation); this is an indication to screen each parent to see if they carry a balanced translocation.

Phenotypic features: foreshortened head (brachycephaly), three fontanelles. The eyes have an upward slant and crescents of skin cover the inner canthi (epicanthic folds); small white spots are situated around the outer third of the iris (Brushfield spots). The nasal bridge is flat and the tongue protuberant and deeply furrowed. A single transverse palmar crease is present on the hand, together with a short, incurved, fifth finger (clinodactyly). A wide gap is present between the first and second toes, often with a longitudinal plantar crease. Hypotonia and delayed development are universal.

Bemberg ME. Genetic factors in disease.
Oxford Textbook of Medicine. Oxford University Press.

Question 5

A. true **B.** false **C.** true **D.** true **E.** true

Apoptosis is a common process during development, adult growth, disease and tissue healing. For example it occurs in the remodelling of neurons during the development of the brain, and in adulthood the cyclic breakdown of the endometrium during menstruation, the death of enterocytes sloughed off the tip of villi during replacement of fresh tissue in the small intestine, and also occurs in pathological processes such as autoimmune disease and cancer.

During apoptosis or programmed cell death, the cell shrinks and becomes denser. There is little or no organelle swelling such as involving mitochondria which can distinguish this process of cell death from ischaemic necrosis where essentially ion-pump failure occurs leading to swelling of the cell prior to rupture. Biochemically, the DNA is broken down into segments that are multiples of around 185 base pairs, due to specific cleavage between nucleosomes. Apoptosis appears to be under genetic control and can be initiated by an internal clock and by external agents in the extracellular compartment such as hormones, cytokines, killer cells and a variety of chemical, physical and viral agents. The time from initiation to final cell destruction is short, of the order of 30 minutes in some cell types. It may be this latter phenomenon that has led to apoptosis becoming recognized only in recent times despite clear histological descriptions even in the nineteenth century. It is important to note that cell suicide may not always occur by apoptosis, cytokine induced cell death may be via apoptosis, that there are several varieties of apoptosis and finally that different cell types may follow different rules. Two of the most prominent extracelular factors activating the process of apoptosis are Fas and Tissue Necrosis Factor (TNF). When Fas binds to its receptor on the cell membrane, a cascade of reactions is triggered by a collection of intracellular cysteine proteases originally called ICE-link enzymes (interleukin 1 beta converting enzyme) which switch on genes that initiate the process of programmed cell death. TNF acts in a similar fashion after interacting with the TNF-1 receptor. The activated apoptotic genes cause the cell to undergo DNA fragmentation, cytoplasmic and chromatin condensation, and eventually membrane bleb formation, with cell breakup and removal of the debris by phagocytes.

Just as proto-oncogenes exist that are responsible for mutations giving rise to oncogenes that have malignant properties, some genes exist that suppress tumour growth the so-called tumour suppressor genes. The most studied of these is the p53 gene on chromosome 17 which triggers apoptosis in normal physiological circumstances. In human cancer p53 genes undergo mutations and the resulting products are unable to slow the cell cycle and thus permit other mutations to DNA to occur. The accumulated mutations eventually cause malignant growth.

Ganong WF. Review of Medical Physiology 1999
19th Edition Appleton and Lange Publishers, Connecticut

Question 6

A. false **B.** true **C.** true **D.** false **E.** true

Tumour necrosis factor (TNF) comprises just one of a long list of important cytokines – some of which are listed below:

Interleukins 1, 2, 4, 6, 10 and 13.
TNF alpha and beta
Interferons (IFN) alpha, beta, and gamma
Colony stimulating factor (IL-3, IL-5)

Chemokines (IL-8), monocyte chemotactic peptide, macrophage inflammatory protein

TNF alpha and beta are involved in cell activation and apoptosis. There are two types: TNF alpha is principally produced by macrophages, TNF beta is secreted mainly by T lymphocytes. TNF is around 17kDa in size; most cells have receptors for it. Whilst not produced in the necrotic centre of tumours it derives its name from its ability to induce haemorrhagic necrosis in experimental tumours. TNF alpha and beta cause fever, hypotension, hypercoagulability and cardiovascular collapse when injected intravenously. They stimulate leucocyte microbiocidal activity, induce adhesion receptors on endothelial cells, and appear to regulate cell growth and apoptosis. TNF alpha may be responsible for the shock syndrome following Gram-negative septicaemia or release of bacterial endotoxin. A low controlled concentration of TNF may be necessary for resistance to infection.

Actions of TNF

1. Treatment of melanoma by limb perfusion (targeting the tumour vasculature).
2. Structurally identical to cachectin previously described as a substance inducing weight loss in animals transplanted with human tumours. The secretion of TNF by macrophages may lead to tuberculomas in post primary TB and the subsequent wasting disease (formerly known as consumption) – characteristic of advanced untreated tuberculosis.
3. TNF and IL-2 produces fever and both may be produced in cancer patients.
4. Cytokines play a major role in the acute phase response. TNF appears to rise before IL-1 and IL-6 and in experimental animals septic shock may be prevented by prior administration of anti-TNF monoclonal or polyclonal antibodies. The characteristic intermittent fever of malaria is associated with the cyclical production of TNF that occurs at schizogony.
5. In studies of the pathogenesis of meningitis TNF induces endothelial cells to secrete nitric oxide, which is a powerful vasodilator – and this may play a role in producing meningococcal shock.
6. In patients with Louse-borne fever treatment with penicillin causes a severe Jarisch-Herxheimer reaction – associated with elevated TNF levels. Treatment with anti-TNF antibodies prior to penicillin prevents this.

Keshav S. Cytokines
Oxford Textbook of Medicine. Oxford University Press.

Question 7

A. false **B.** true **C.** true **D.** false **E.** true

Anatomy of the sympathetic system: the cell bodies of the preganglionic neurons unlike those of the parasympathetic system lie within the spinal cord and exit via the thoracic and upper lumbar nerves to synapse in the peripheral sympathetic ganglia running in the paraspinal chain. The exception to the rule is the adrenal medulla, which is innervated directly by preganglionic fibres passing through the splanchnic nerves to synapse directly with secretory cells that secret catecholamines (mainly adrenaline). Sympathetic fibres from the right stellate ganglion are distributed mainly to the sinus node and the right atrium and ventricle whilst in the left, the ventrolateral cardiac nerve provides a major sympathetic supply to the left atrium and posterior and lateral surfaces of the left ventricle.

Noradrenaline (NAd) is the natural transmitter that is stored in neurosecretory granules in sympathetic nerve terminals. Depolarisation causes release of intraneuronal calcium, migration of the granules to the neuronal membrane, release of NAd into the synaptic cleft and activation of postsynaptic receptors. NAds action is controlled by neuronal uptake, on the presynaptic terminal (re-uptake), broken down by catechol-O-methyl-transferase or diffuses away into the circulation. Many adrenergic receptors exist.

Receptor	***Action on circulation***
Alpha -1	vasoconstriction (increase in contractility)
Alpha -2	vasoconstriction presynaptic sympathetic inhibition
Beta -1	increase in heart rate (sinus node) increase in contractility (atrium, ventricle) increase in conduction (AV node)
Beta -2	vasodilatation (bronchodilation)
Dopaminergic-1	renal and mesenteric vasodilatation
Dopaminergic-2	vasodilatation

Adrenergic receptor activity of endogenous and synthetic catecholamines

Catecholamines	***Receptor subtype***					
	alpha-1	–2	beta-1	–2	DA-1	DA-2
Dopamine	++	+	++	0	+++	++
NAd	+++	++	+++	+/–	0	0
Ad	++	++	+++	+++	0	0
Isoprenaline	0	0	+++	++	0	0
Dobutamine	+	+/–	+++	++	0	0
Salbutamol	0	0	+	+++	0	0
Dopexamine	0	0	+	++	++	+

Interaction with alpha receptors appears to increase cytoplasmic calcium whereas stimulation of the beta receptor stimulates a rise in intracellular cAMP.

Forfar JC. Catecholamines and the sympathetic nervous system. Oxford Textbook of Medicine. Oxford University Press.

Question 8

A. false **B.** true **C.** false **D.** false **E.** true

Afferent pathways to the brainstem for the pupillary light reflex are as follows:

1. light impinges on the back of the retina
2. impulses are carried from the optic nerve through the optic chiasm to the lateral geniculate nucleus
3. these fibres pass to the pretectal nucleus in the midbrain
4. synaptic fibres then pass to the ipsilateral and contralateral Edinger Westphal nucleus
5. from here fibres travel in the third nerve from the midbrain to the ciliary ganglion
6. and postganglionic fibres pass from here to innervate the iris and ciliary muscles

The light reflex will be diminished if:

corneal opacities /cataracts are present
lesions of optic nerve, chiasm or optic tract exist
local disease of the eye e.g. iridocyclitis may cause adhesions preventing pupillary constriction
lesion of IIIrd nerve nucleus, IIIrd nerve, the ciliary ganglion or short ciliary nerves

Causes of a small pupil:
Horner's
Argyll Robertson pupil
Myotonic dystrophy
Pontine lesions
Acute iritis
Opiates
Organophosphate poisoning

Causes of a large pupil:
IIIrd nerve palsy
Holmes Adie Pupil
Midbrain lesion
Congenital syphilis
Local trauma
Anticholinergics / benzodiazepines / cocaine / mydriatics

Scadding JW, Gibby J. Neurological disease
Oxford Textbook of Medicine. Oxford University Press.

Question 9

A. true **B.** false **C.** true **D.** true **E.** false

Anatomy of the VIIth nerve

The VIIth cranial nerve has its nucleus in the pons; the nerve emerges from the pons and medulla medial to the VIIIth nerve in the cerebello-pontine angle. It enters the internal auditory canal with the VIIIth nerve and passes to the geniculate ganglion. Apart from a small offshoot (the greater petrosal nerve – motor to the lacrimial gland) the main part of the nerve enters the facial canal giving off fibres to:

1. the chorda tympani (taste)
2. a branch to the stapedius

before it leaves the skull through the stylomastoid foramen (facial muscles / salivary glands). The taste fibres from the anterior 2/3 of the tongue pass through the lingual nerve and join the facial nerve via the chorda tympani; their cell bodies are in the geniculate ganglion.

Scadding JW, Gibby J. Neurological disease
Oxford Textbook of Medicine. Oxford University Press.

Question 10

A. true **B.** false **C.** true **D.** false **E.** false

21-hydroxylase deficiency is inherited as a recessive condition. The disease is due to a mutation or deletion of the gene for 21-hydroxylase, located in chromosome 6. The incidence is rare (1 in 15,000 births). The severe classic form can be recognized in newborn girls by ambiguous external genitalia caused by high levels of adrenal androgens. 75% of affected newborn babies develop severe mineralocorticoid deficiency and salt loss. Male infants are normally virilized. Affected males present as salt losing with acute adrenal insufficiency and sodium and water depletion, usually within the first weeks of life.

In Figure 1 the flow diagram depicts the steroid pathways in the adrenal zona glomerulosa, fasciculata and reticularis, (ovary and testes not shown for brevity). 21-alpha-hydroxylase acts at a) and 11-beta-hyroxylase acts at b). The balance of steroids secreted is determined by the enzymes present (represented by arrows).

Mortality is higher than in males. Non salt losing males will present with accelerated growth and sexual development but small testes (sexual precocity and pseudopuberty) and later, with azospermia. Diagnosis is made by showing raised levels of plasma / salivary / urinary levels of 17-alpha- hydroxyprogesterone.

Wheetman AP, McLean DC Endocrinology. In: Medicine Souhami/Moxham (eds) Churchill Livinsgstone

Figure 1. The steroid pathways in the adrenal zona glomerulosa, fasciculata and reticularis, (ovary and testes not shown for brevity). 21-α-hydroxylase acts at a) and 11-β-hyroxylase acts at b). The balance of steroids secreted is determined by the enzymes present (represented by arrows).

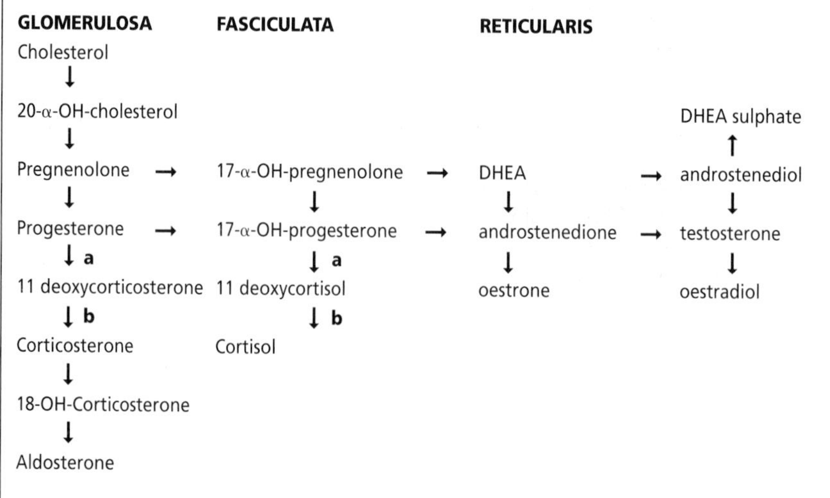

Question 11

A. false **B.** false **C.** true **D.** true **E.** false

Adult haemoglobin (HbA) is a tetramer of two alpha and two beta chains. Each globin chain has 1 haem molecule. At high oxygen tensions in the lungs oxygen is rapidly taken up and can be released easily at lower tensions in the tissues. When one haem molecule takes on oxygen the affinity for oxygen of the remaining haems of the tetramer increases markedly. Oxygen affinity is decreased by:

1. increasing CO_2 tensions (Bohr effect) which facilitates O_2 transfer to the tissues
2. decreased pH (caused by CO_2 influx).

CO_2 acts in two ways: firstly by passing into the red cells where carbonic anhydrase produces carbonic acid (decreasing the pH) and secondly by combining with the terminal amino acid groups to form carbamino compounds. O_2 affinity is also decreased by 2,3,-diphosphoglycerate (DPG) which shifts the O_2 dissociation curve to the right and by increasing body temperature i.e. a state of reduced O_2 affinity.

Causes of increased DPG (increased P50, reduced whole blood O_2 affinity)
Anaemia
Alkalosis
Hyperphosphataemia
Renal failure
Hypoxia
Pregnancy
Cyanotic congenital heart disease
Thyrotoxicosis
Some red cell enzyme deficiency

Cause of decreased DPG (increased whole blood O_2 affinity)
Acidosis
Cardiogenic or septicaemic shock
Hypophosphataemia
Hypothyroidism
Hypopituitarism
Following replacement with stored blood

Weatherall J. Anaemia: pathophysiology, classification and clinical features Oxford Textbook of Medicine. Oxford University Press.

Question 12

A. true **B**. false **C**. true **D**. false **E**. false

The immune system is an organization of cells and molecules with specialized roles in defending against infection. There are two fundamentally different types of responses to invading microbes: the innate response and the acquired (adaptive) response. Two major differences exist between the two: the first is the specificity of the acquired/immune response e.g. the antibody response is a good example of this although it also occurs in the cellular immune response. The second is memory: innate (natural) responses occur to the same extent however many times the infectious agent is encountered, whereas acquired (adaptive) responses improve on repeated exposure to a given infection.

The innate responses use phagocytic cells (neutrophils, monocytes, and macrophages), cells that release inflammatory mediators (basophils, mast cells, and eosinophils), and natural killer cells. The molecular components of innate responses include complement, acute-phase proteins, and cytokines such as the interferons. Acquired responses involve the proliferation of antigen-specific B and T cells, which occurs when the surface receptors of these cells bind to antigen. Specialized cells, called antigen-presenting cells, display the antigen to lymphocytes and collaborate with them in the response to the antigen. B cells secrete immunoglobulins, the antigen-specific antibodies responsible for eliminating extracellular microorganisms. T cells help B cells to make antibody and can also eradicate intracellular pathogens by activating macrophages and by killing virally infected cells. Innate and acquired responses usually work together to eliminate pathogens.

Mediators of allergic reactions

Mediator	***Cell source***	***Target Tissue***
Histamine	mast cells, basophils,	(relaxation of) vascular smooth muscle (contraction of) non-vascular smooth muscle
Eicosanoids		
Prostaglandins	platelets	vascular smooth muscle bronchial smooth muscle
Leukotrienes	basophils, eosinophils	vascular smooth muscle, mucous glands
Thromboxane	neutrophils/mast cell	vascular/non vascular smooth muscle

Platelet activating factors	mast cells/basophils	bronchi/vascular smooth muscle
Heparin	mast cells	platelets
Chemokines	macrophages, lymphocytes mast cells	chemoattraction
Kallikrein	basophil	vascular smooth muscle
Hageman factor	basophil	vascular smooth muscle

Eicosanoids are synthesized by mast cells, basophils, and eosinophils through the oxygenation of arachidonic acid metabolites via two pathways: the cyclo-oxygenase pathway forms prostaglandins (PG) and thromboxanes and the 5-lipoxygenase pathway generates leukotrienes (LT). PGD2 and thromboxane A2 are bronchoconstrictors in asthma. The leukotrienes induce increased systemic vascular permeability, smooth-muscle contraction, and mucus secretion.

McMichael AJ. Principles of Immunology
Oxford Textbook of Medicine. Oxford University Press.

Question 13

A. false **B.** true **C.** true **D.** false **E.** false

Vertical transmission of human immunodeficiency virus (HIV), from mother to infant, can occur in utero, during delivery and by breast milk. Rates of vertical transmission appear to be much higher in developing countries and may be about 30%. It is unclear how much of the excess can be attributed to breast feeding and what advice should be given to seropositive mothers. For infants in poor families the risk of dying through the inappropriate use of formula milk may exceed the risk of acquiring HIV from breast milk. In comparison to industrialized nations where the health care system is better early in the course of the disease high grade pathogens can cause disease such as mycobacterium tuberculosis, Streptococcal pneumonia, varicella zoster virus and the presentation may be typical for that disease such as typical primary TB, lobar pneumonia, and dermatological shingles. Only as the HIV progresses do clinical features of the underlying immunosuppression such as oral candidiasis, leukoplakia, fungal skin rashes, zoster scar or unexplained weight loss occur. The AIDS-related complex is the pre-AIDS phase of HIV disease. High-grade pathogens still predominate but others now include salmonellae, Eschericia coli, shigella and staphylococcus aureus. Mixed infections are now being recognized.

Diseases diagnostic of AIDS without the laboratory evidence of HIV:

candidiasis: oesophageal, pulmonary
crytococcus: extrapulmonary
cryptosporidiosis: diarrhoea persisting for longer than 1 month
Herpes simplex
primary cerebral lymphoma
lymphoid interstitial pneumonia
mycobacterium avium
mycobacterium kansasii
progressive multifocal leucoencephalopathy
cerebral toxoplasmosis

Major modes of transmission will be well know to you:

perinatal (vertical)
sexual (anal / vaginal intercourse)
sharing of contaminated needles
transfusions of infected blood and blood products (especially infusion of infected factor VIII)

WHO estimates for the year 2000 are that 40 million will be infected worldwide. 90% of these will be in developing countries in sub Saharan Africa, South and South east Asia, Latin America, and the Caribbean. Patterns of infection

Pattern 1: USA / Europe / Australia and New Zealand homosexual men / injecting drug users
By the end of 1991 in southern Europe there were more cases through injecting drug users than in homosexual and bisexual men.

Pattern 2: Sub Saharan Africa / Caribbean
Predominantly heterosexual / perinatal
Male to female ratio 1:1

Pattern 3: North Africa / Middle East / Eastern Europe / Asia + Oceania
(other than Australia and New Zealand).
Late epidemics: therefore figures are less accurate.
Increasing prevalence in IV drug abusers and prostitutes.

Weller IVD et al. HIV infection and AIDS.
Oxford Textbook of Medicine. Oxford University Press.

Question 14

A. true **B.** false **C.** true **D.** true **E.** false

Clinical aspects of Epstein-Barr virus (EBV) infection (mononucleosis-like syndrome):

Affects mainly adolescents
Pharyngitis/tonsilitis prominent
Palatine petechiae characteristic
Fever
Cervical lymphadenopathy (tender)
Splenomegaly
Lymphocytosis 90% of cases
Abnormal liver functions tests 90% (jaundice in 5–10% of cases)
Characteristic rash if exposed to ampicillin in 90% of cases

Less common complications of EBV infection include:

haemolytic anemia
thrombocytopenia
aplastic anemia
myocarditis
hepatitis
genital ulcers
splenic rupture
rash
neurologic complications such as Guillain–Barré syndrome,encephalitis,and meningitis.

Viruses implicated in tumour origins:

Epstein Barr virus	Burkitt's lymphoma nasopharyngeal carcinoma cerebral lymphoma (when immunocompromised) eg in organ transplant patients X-linked lymphoproliferative syndrome (Duncans disease) Hodgkins lymphoma lethal midline granuloma (T cell NHL) gastric cancer
Hepatitis B and C	hepatocellular carcinoma
Papillomavirus (HPV) serotypes 16 and 18	squamous cell carcinoma (SCC) of the cervix penile, vulval and anal carcinomas (SCC)
HTLV 1 and II	T cell leukaemia/lymphoma
HHV-8	Kaposis sarcoma

Cohen JI. EBV infection.
NEJM 2000 343: 7; 481–492

Question 15

A. true **B.** false **C.** false **D.** true **E.** true

Viral encephalitis is infection of the brain parenchyma and can occur rarely through some common viral infections such as:

Herpes simplex virus
EpsteinBarr virus
Cytomegalovirus
Varicella-zoster virus
Human herpesvirus 6
Non-polio enteroviruses
Tick-borne encephalitis
Mumps virus
Rabies virus

The mortality may be high and even for those who survive there may be long term neurological deficits. Infection may occur at any time from the neo-natal period to old age involving primary infection and also reactivation of latent virus. In the UK it is a notifiable disease. CNS infections may occur through a neuronal route eg rabies or herpes simplex virus or a haematogenous route eg tick or mosquito bite. In the case of neuronal infection the virus enters through retrograde axoplasmic flow directly into the brain.

Typically encephalitis is acute with fever, headache and disturbances in higher mental function (e.g. confusion, delirium, behaviour changes, dysphasia / aphasia, temporal lobe seizures, focal neurological signs proceeding to coma). The most common and most important encephalitis is with Herpes simplex virus (HSV). The incidence is around 1/250,000–500,000/year with 1/3 cases in young people under 20, 1/2 in those over 50. In 2/3 of cases the aetiology is through viral reactivation. Primary infection does occur but mainly in neonates. Most patients do not have a cold sore. HSV primarily targets the temporal lobes and being cytolytic causes destruction of nervous tissue in this area. The site of replication can be recognized by the subsequent symptoms: temporal lobe seizures, speech disorders, personality changes and altered behaviour.

In the history it is important to elicit any details of recent travel that may suggest a specific virus eg. rabies, Japanese and tick-borne encephalitis, the recently discovered Nipah and Hendra arthropod-borne viruses from Singapore and Malaysia, and West Nile fever, which is now endemic in New York and New England, USA. It is imperative to look for evidence of immunocompromise which may suggest a slightly different group of viruses such as CMV, Varicella Zoster virus, HIV, EBV and JC virus.

Diagnosis is by lumbar puncture though many patients may require a CT head (especially if HSV encephalitis is considered) to rule out evidence of raised intracranial pressure. Typical CSF findings are similar to that of viral meningitis ie

pleocytosis
mildly elevated protein (0.5–1.0 g/litre)
normal CSF:blood glucose ratio
the cell count reveals predominantly lymphocytes
If in the first 24 hours: neutrophil predominance

With the Polymerase chain reaction (PCR) analysis – diagnosis of viral meningitis and encephalitis has been transformed and has made brain biopsy almost obsolete in the diagnosis of herpes simplex encephalitis. As few as ten copies of a nucleic acid sequence can be detected and has almost replaced conventional cell culture because it is more sensitive.

Management in the early stages of suspected encephalitis includes: PCR analysis, cell culture, throat swabs, stool and vesicular fluid or lesion swabs, clotted blood for seroconversion (HIV/HSV/Mumps IgM) and antibiotics until viral meningitis or encephalitis is confirmed and/or bacterial meningitis is excluded. For HSV encephalitis high dose aciclovir should be started early, although this drug has transformed the outlook from very poor to moderate the mortalitiy is still 50% at 2 years. Good prognositic signs in HSV encephalitis include aciclovir within 4 days and a GCS over 6 at the outset.

Rice P. Viral meningitis and encephalitis
Medicine 2001 29: 2; 54–57.

Question 16

A. false **B.** false **C.** true **D.** false **E.** false

Clostridia tetanus is one of several clostridial species such as C. perfringens, C. botulinum and C. difficile. As a species they are anaerobic Gram-positive rods which form spores that enhance their survival and they are difficult to destroy by disinfection and sterilization. Spores may be found in a variety of places such as soil and the normal flora of the human intestine. C. tetanus that finds its way into an open wound eg a trivial thorn injury and subsequent work with soil handling may lead to the condition called tetanus. Following germination of the spores a neurotoxin called tetanospasmin is released that blocks only inhibitory synapses on CNS motor neurones leading to uninhibited excitation and therefore muscle spasm. The toxin may travel from the site of infection up the nerve causing local tetanus before spreading via the blood stream to the CNS proper. As cranial nerves are generally short they are affected first hence the famous presentation of lock jaw. In the UK the incidence has fallen with the introduction of antibiotics, vaccination and prophylaxis for open wounds. Over a ten year period (1989–1999) 14 deaths were recorded out of a total 80 cases. Over 50% of cases occur in patients over 65. The diagnosis is often made clinically and investigations should include a tissue sample if possible or a swab of the wound for gram staining and anaerobic culture. A gardening injury 2–3 weeks earlier is a good example of a scenario leading to tetanus: often there is no obvious adverse reaction at the wound site in terms of pus or rash and swabs from this site may be negative for C. tetanus.

For children immunization should take place with three doses of tetanus toxoid and a booster at 10 years – a second booster at the next 10 year interval should confer life long immunity. For any open wound prophylaxis should be given unless a booster has been given within 10 years. If no booster has been given immediate cover is only conferred with human tetanus immunoglobulin in addition to tetanus toxoid.

For confirmed cases of tetanus management should include:

1. Anti-tetanus immunoglobulin and penicillin
2. Intensive care admission with a view if required to sedation, ventilation and care to intercurrent infections, line bacteraemia and deep vein thrombosis
3. Vaccination following the acute illnes as no immunity is conferred

Duerdin BI, Brazier JS. Tetanus and other Clostridial diseases Medicine 2001 29: 3; 93–95

Question 17

A. false **B.** false **C.** true **D.** false **E.** true

Giardia intestinalis (syn. G. lamblia) is a protozoal illnes commonly encountered by travellers to endemic areas. It is also seen in children in day care centres and those with immunoglobulin deficiency states. It commonly resides in the gut lumen: the trophoziote is found predominantly in the proximal small intestine. Many pathogenic mechanisms have been proposed for its mechanism of action including partial villus atrophy which can been seen at endoscopy and subequent histology on duodenal biopsies, microvillous disruption, mucosal inflammation, inhibition of pancreatic enzyme activity and alteration in bile salt metabolism. For anyone with a strong clinical history suggestive of Giardiasis the investigations should be as follows: stool specimens x3 for ova cysts and parasites looking specifically for cysts (found typically in over 75% of cases) and if negative, gastroscopy and duodenal biopsy and/or aspiration. Stool specimens can be on unstained faeces or stained with Lugols iodine which stains cysts brown. Recently tests such as enzyme linked immunosorbent assays are now available for stool specimens to detect faecal antigens. First line treatment is generally with metronidazole or tinidazole; second line includes albendazole or mepacrine.

Farthing MJG and Kelly P. Protozoal gastrointestinal infections. Medince 2001 29: 2; 72–74

Question 18

A. true **B.** true **C.** false **D.** true **E.** false

The porphyrias are a group of in born errors of metabolism caused by an abnormality in the enzymes involved in the production of haem. There is a build up in the intermediate components called porphyrins. The resulting chemical and clinical abnormalities are dictated by the specific enzyme abnormality in the pathway. They either cause a build up in hepatic or bone marrow porphyrins. Acute intermittent porphyria is autosomal dominant and associated with abdominal pain and neuropsychiatric symptoms. It is a cause of dark urine and it can be precipitated by many drugs including oestrogens and barbiturates. Symptoms are caused by accumulation of delta laevulinic acid. Porphyria cutanea tarda is associated with photosensitivity and hirsutism and is a common finding in alcoholics. It causes a bullous skin eruption in sun-exposed areas that heal by scarring. Diagnosis is by an elevated urinary uroporphyrin and treatment is with venesection.

Acute Porphyrias	***Biochemical and clinical manifestations***
1. Acute intermittent porphyria	1, 2 and 3: increased porphyrin precursors
2. Variegate porphyria	1, 2 and 3: acute neurovisceral attacks
3. Hereditary coproporphyria	2 and 3: increased porphyrins
	2 and 3: cutaneous photosensitivity
	all acutes are Autosomal Dominant
	all are often precipitated by drugs
	all are potentially life threatening

Other precipitants of acute porphyria: alcohol, fasting, hormones and infection. Safe drugs in porphyria: aspirin, paracetamol, codeine, penicillin, low-dose chloroquine, chlorpromazine, metoclopramide, sodium valproate, propranolol, labetalol, digoxin and insulin.

Non-acute porphyrias

4. Porphyria cutanea tarda	4, 5 and 6: increased porphyrins
5. Erythropoietic protoporphyria	4, 5 and 6: cutaneous photosensitivity
6. Congenital porphyria	

Increased excretion of circulating porphyrins is found in a number of other diseases, either because the synthesis of haem is disturbed or because the mechanism of excretion is abnormal. The most important of these are lead poisoning, iron-deficiency anaemia, and alcohol ingestion, although there is a heterogenous group of other diseases in which porphyrin metabolism is deranged.

Causes of abnormalities of haem synthesis: iron deficiency anaemia, lead poisoning, alcohol induced sideroblastic anaemia, other causes of sideroblastic anaemia.

McColl KEL et al. Porphyrin metabolism and the porphyrias Oxford Textbook of Medicine. Oxford University Press.

Question 19

A. true **B.** true **C.** false **D.** true **E.** true

An increase in red cell mass can be classified as either primary [polycythaemia rubra vera (PRV)] or secondary. PRV is a myeloproliferative disorder that is characterized by a stem cell disorder.

Secondary causes can be further divided into hypoxic causes or due to inappropriate increase in erythropoiesis.

HYPOXIC CAUSES
Living at high altitude
Cardiovascular disease especially if there is a right to left shunt
Respiratory disease
Heavy smoking
Pickwickian syndrome
Methaemoglobinaemia

DUE TO INAPPROPRIATE INCREASE IN ERYTHROPOIESIS
Renal disease esp. Wilm's tumours
Hepatocellular carcinoma
Adrenal tumours
Massive uterine fibroids
Cerebellar haemangioblastoma

There may be an apparent increase in red cell mass. This occurs when there is normal red cell volume but decrease plasma volume. This can occur in stress (known as the Gaisbock Syndrome), dehydration and burns.

Weatherall DJ. The relative and secondary polycythaemias. Oxford Textbook of Medicine. Oxford University Press.

Question 20

A. false **B.** false **C.** true **D.** true **E.** false

Hereditary spherocytosis is the commonest haemolytic anaemia in Europeans. It is a condition in which there is a defect in red cell membranes through a deficiency in a structural protein called spectrin. Spherocytes are more rigid than normal red cells and hence are less pliable (increased fragility) therefore passage through the microcirculation within the spleen leads to preferential trapping in the cords and removal from the circulation. Although it occurs in most races it is especially common in northern Europeans with a prevalence of around 1:5000. It has two patterns of inheritance: 75% autosomal inheritance, 25% non-dominant (probably autosomal recessive). Clinically it may present with neonatal jaundice, anaemia, splenomegaly and leg ulcers and may even be asymptomatic. Diagnosis is aided by examination of the blood film and/or red cell fragility tests. There will be evidence of haemolytic anaemia (increased bilirubin, decreased haptoglobins and raised urinary urobilinogen).

Complications include:

aplastic crisis especially with parvovirus B19
megaloblastic anaemia secondary to folate deficiency
increased level of haemolysis with intercurrent illness
gall stones
extramedullary haemopoiesis
iron overload secondary to multiple transfusions

Treatment is by splenectomy. Any planned splenectomy should be proceeded by vaccination against pneumococcal, haemophilus and probably meningococcal infections. Patients should also have prophylactic antibiotics (probably lifelong).

Ever SW, Lux SE. Genetic disorders of the red-cell membrane. Oxford Textbook of Medicine. Oxford University Press.

Question 21

A. true **B.** true **C.** false **D.** true **E.** true

There are many drugs that cause haemolytic anaemia but here are some of the college favourites:

Antimalarials
Arsenic
Dapsone
High dose penicillin
Lead
Methyldopa
Phenacetin
Snake venoms
Sulphonamides

Others cause haemolysis in the presence of other abnormalities such as G6PD deficiency. In practice always check the British National Formulary when treating patients with abnormalities such as porphyria or G6PD deficiency.

J.L. Burton and C.J. Healey Aids to Postgraduate medicine
Sixth edition Churchill Livingstone 1994

Provan D, Chisholm M, Duncombe A, Singer C, Smith A
Oxford Handbook of Clinical Haematology Oxford University Press 1998

Question 22

A. true **B.** false **C.** false **D.** true **E.** true

Questions are commonly asked about prescribing during pregnancy.

In the first trimester ie up to 16 weeks the concern is that drugs may exert a teratogenic affect on the foetus.

The following are examples:

Warfarin is associated with cartilage and long bone problems
Lithium is associated with cardiac abnormalities

Sodium valproate and retinoids give rise to neural tube defects.
Phenytoin is associated with cleft lip or palate

Later on in pregnancy drugs may cross the placenta and exert an effect on the foetus. Examples of this include:

Gentamicin causing VIIIth nerve damage and hence deafness
Carbimazole leading to a neonatal goitre
Tetracyclines causing dental discolouration
Sulphonamides may cause jaundice kernicterus
Warfarin is associated with fetal and neonatal haemorrhages
Alcohol and narcotics can give rise to CNS depression and withdrawal syndromes.

NSAID's can cause premature closure of the fetal ductus arteriosus, delayed labour and increased blood loss.

Sulphonylureas are known to cause fetal and neonatal hypoglycaemia

British National Formulary
BMA and Royal Pharmaceutical Society of Great Britain

Koren G, Pastusza. A, Ito S Drug Therapy: Drugs in Pregnancy
NEJM 1998 338(16): 1128–1137

Question 23

A. true **B.** false **C.** true **D.** true **E.** true

Cimetidine inhibits hepatic enzymes. Phenytoin is metabolized in the liver and so co-administration may lead to an increase in phenytoin levels. Phenytoin has a narrow therapeutic window and even a small increase may lead to increased side effects or toxicity. Phenelzine is a monoamine oxidase inhibitor (MAOI). L dopa releases stores of monoamines that cannot be broken down in the presence of a MAOI and may precipitate a hypertensive crisis. Amiloride acts on the distal tubule preventing potassium secretion in exchange for sodium. There is an increased risk of nephrotoxicity with NSAIDs and they may antagonize the diuretic effect. Verapamil is a class IV antiarrhythmic. It acts by decreasing AV nodal conduction. It can potentiate the negative effects of beta-blockers at the AV node.

Commonly used antiarrhythmic drugs

Class Ia	Quinidine Disopyramide Procainamide

Class Ib	Lignocaine Mexiletine
Class Ic	Flecainide
Class II	Beta-blockers eg. Atenolol
Class III	Sotalol Amiodarone
Class IV	Verapamil Digoxin Adenosine

Cobbe SM, Rankin AC. Cardiac Arrhythmias
Oxford Textbook of Medicine. Oxford University Press.

Question 24

A. false **B.** true **C.** true **D.** true **E.** false

The following are drugs that induce hepatic enzymes

Phenytoin
Carbamazepine
Barbiturates
Rifampicin
Alcohol (chronic use)
Griseofulvin
Sulphonylureas
Mnemonic: PCBRAGS

The following inhibit liver enzymes

Omeprazole
Disulfiram
Erythromycin
Valproate
Isoniazid
Ciprofloxacin, cimetidine
Ethanol (acute)
Sulphonamides
Mnemonic: ODEVICES

Meyer UA. Overview of Enzymes of Drug Metabolism
Journal Of Pharmacokinetic Biopharm 1996 24(5): 449–59

Question 25

A. false **B.** true **C.** true **D.** true **E.** true

Metronidazole is reduced to a substance that interacts with DNA to cause a loss of helical DNA structure and strand breakage resulting in the inhibition of protein synthesis and cell death in susceptible organisms. It is well absorbed orally, intravenously and rectally. It can cause a metallic taste and a disulfiram type reaction with alcohol. Prolonged use is associated with peripheral neuropathy. Incidences where its prescription must be made with care include hepatic failure, pregnancy and breast feeding.

British National Formulary
BMA and Royal Pharmaceutical Society of Great Britain

Question 26

A. true **B.** false **C.** true **D.** false **E.** true

Isotretinoin is a useful treatment in comedonal acne. It requires several months of treatment. It causes an increase in plasma lipids and monitoring should be undertaken during treatment with a check every 3 months.

Side effects include:

dry eyes and hence increased risk of keratitis
dry nasal mucosa
optic neuritis
photophobia
benign intracranial hypertension
myalgia
anaemia

Isotretinoin is therefore a toxic drug which should only be used under the supervision of a dermatologist. In addition it is associated with fetal abnormalities and should not be given to women of child bearing years unless effective contraception is undertaken for 1 month prior, during and 1 month after treatment.

British National Formulary
BMA and Royal Pharmaceutical Society of Great Britain

Question 27

A. true **B.** false **C.** true **D.** true **E.** true

The Cholesterol and Recurrent Events (CARE) study showed that treatment with an HMG CoA reductase inhibitor decreased the incidence in coronary events after non fatal MI and cardiac deaths even in people with average cholesterol levels. It has been shown that they slow the progression of atherosclerosis and decreases the risk of cardiovascular events and mortality.

Their side effects include

rhabdomyolysis
altered liver function tests and rarely hepatitis
headache
abdominal pain, nausea and diarrhoea

Sacks FM, Pfeffer MA, More et al The effect of pravastatin on coronary events after MI in patients with average cholesterol. NEJM 1996: 335;14: 1001–1006

Question 28

A. true **B.** true **C.** true **D.** false **E.** true

In the context of poisoning haemodialysis is useful for overdoses with the following:

Lithium
barbiturates
alcohol
methanol
ethylene glycol
salicylates

Charcoal haemoperfusion is used for:

paracetamol
theophylline
short acting barbiturates

Activated charcoal causes decreased absorption from the GI tract of many drugs. It is given in repeated doses with overdoses of:

carbamazepine
dapsone
phenobarbitone
quinine
theophylline

Theophylline causes hypokalaemia by two mechanisms in overdose. First by induced vomiting, second by intracellular movement of potassium. In addition arrhythmias may be precipitated by inhibiting phosphodiesterase.

Ethylene glycol is the active constituent of anti freeze. Patients who have drunk it may appear similar to those with alcohol intoxication, but they do not smell of alcohol. It is broken down to oxalate which causes an increased anion gap metabolic acidosis.

Other causes of an increased anionic gap acidosis are

lactic acidosis
ketoacidosis
renal failure
hepatic failure
aspirin
methanol
The anion gap is calculated by (Na +K) – (Cl + HCO3)

Quinine is very toxic in overdose. It can cause blindness, tinnitus and headaches. Seek advice from the poisons centre.

Meredith TJ et al. Introduction and epidemiology of poisoning
Oxford Textbook of Medicine. Oxford University Press.

Question 29

A. false **B.** false **C.** false **D.** true **E.** false

The student t test is a parametric test. It assumes data is normally distributed.

In this test $p > 0.05$, the accepted value of statistical significance. This means that the outcome could have occurred by chance in more than 1 in 20. It has not reached statistical significance and so the null hypothesis is accepted, ie no difference between the 2 groups. This is only a measure of statistical significance not clinical significance.

Confidence levels are a measure of how sure one is that the true mean lies within the interval. The interval is calculated by taking the mean + and – the standard error of the mean. This means that one is 95% confident that the true mean lies within this interval.

Driscoll P et al. An introduction to everyday statistics–1
J Accid Emerg Med 2000 17: 205–211

Swinscow TDV. Statistics at Square One
Published by the British Medical Journal

Paper 1 Answers

Question 30

A. true **B.** true **C.** false **D.** false **E.** true

Osteoporosis is a condition in which there is reduced bone mass with normal mineralization. It is defined by the World Health Organization as a T score of less than or equal to –2.5 measured on bone densitometry.

Risk factors are:

female sex
increasing age
menopause <45 years
hypogonadism
family history especially if the mother had a hip fracture
smoking
high alcohol intake
sedentary lifestyle
previous fractures
steroid treatment

Medical conditions such as Cushing's syndrome, hyperthyroidism, hyperparathyroidism, chronic renal failure, scurvy

Certain treatments (or lack of): heparin infusion, poor calcium intake, and cyclosporin treatment

Ulcerative colitis and Crohns disease

Nulliparity

Rare associations are osteogenesis imperfecta, glycogen storage disease, childhood cirrhosis, and systemic mastocytosis.

Wilkin TJ. Changing perceptions in osteoporosis
BMJ vol 318(7187) 27 March 1999 862–864

Christiansen C. Skeletal osteoporosis
Journal of Bone and Mineral Research. 8 Suppl 2: S475–80, Dec 1993

Question 31

A. true **B.** true **C.** true **D.** false **E.** false

SLE is a multisystem inflammatory connective tissue disease which is essentially a small vessel vasculitis with non organ specific autoantibodies. It usually presents between age 16 and 55. The female:male ratio is 10:1. It is more common and more severe in

Asians and West Indians and rarely occurs in black Africans. The American College of Rheumatology has a revised classification for SLE. When 4 or more of the following are present then it is strongly suggestive of a diagnosis of SLE

malar rash
discoid lupus
photosensitivity
oral ulceration
non erosive arthritis of 2 or more joints
serositis – pleurisy or pericarditis
proteinuria
psychosis or fits
haematological disorder – haemolytic anaemia, thrombocytopenia, leucopenia, lymphopenia
ANA
Immunological disorder – LE cells, anti-dsDNA antibody, false positive VDRL

More than 95% of patients are ANA positive. Less than 50% have anti double stranded DNA antibodies. Complement deficiencies can occur and C3 and C4 are useful monitors of disease activity. C4 is part of the classical pathway and C3 is common to both pathways. A small number of babies born to mothers with SLE have neonatal lupus. This appears to be limited to women who are anti Ro or anti La positive. The neonates may have a self-limiting rash. It is associated with congenital heart block in which there is fibrosis of the conduction system. The block is usually permanent.

A drug induced lupus type syndrome is well recognized. This is more common in men than women. CNS and renal involvement is rare. Patients are often anti histone positive. Drugs implicated are procainamide, hydralazine and isoniazid.

Frances C Hall and Mark J Walport
Medicine 1998 26;4:5–12
Michael Snaith. ABC of Rheumatology
BMJ Publishing group 3rd ed 1997

Question 32

A. true **B.** false **C.** true **D.** true **E.** false

Atrial septal defects (ASD) result from failure of fusion of either the septum primum or septum secundum with the endocardial cushions during the first trimester of foetal growth. Primum atrial septal defects are the more serious being classified as partial or complete

AV canal lesions depending on the absence or presence of an associated VSD component. They usually present in infancy or childhood with over half requiring surgery before the age of ten. Characteristic ECG changes include right bundle branch block (RBBB), left axis deviation (LAD), long PR interval, and conduction defects. Primum ASDs are associated with Down's syndrome, Klinefelter's syndrome, and Noonan's syndrome.

Secundum atrial septal defects account for the majority of cases and commonly remain asymptomatic until adulthood with many only being diagnosed after the fourth or fifth decade. Symptoms associated with them include atrial dysrythmias, especially atrial fibrillation, cardiac failure, shunt reversal with the development of Eisenmenger's syndrome, and paradoxical embolisation. Clinically right heart signs predominate in association with a pulmonary flow murmur and fixed splitting of the second heart sound. ECG changes are partial or complete RBBB with RAD. Surgical closure is recommended if the right-to-left shunt is 2:1 or more at cardiac catheterisation. Patients with a history of secundum ASD closure may develop mitral regurgitation many years later due to an associated floppy mitral valve.

Swanton RH. Cardiology 4th Ed. Blackwell Scientific Publications Ltd. Oxford

Question 33

A. false **B.** false **C.** true **D.** false **E.** false

There have now been six major studies addressing the use of oral anticoagulants and anti-platelet agents in the primary and secondary prevention of stroke in patients with non-rheumatic atrial fibrillation. In primary prevention warfarin therapy reduced the risk of stroke from 5% to 1.3% a year and mortality by one third. With secondary prevention in patients who have suffered a previous stroke or TIA the risk of recurrent stroke is reduced from 12% a year to 5%. The maximum decrease in risk of stroke occurs when the INR target range is 2.0 -3.0. An INR >3.0 is associated with a markedly increased risk of intracranial hemorrhage. Aspirin resulted in a 36% reduction in stroke, making it approximately half as effective as warfarin.

Antithrombotic prophylaxis should be determined by clinical risk classification. Echocardiography may add additional information in marginal cases.

Patients who have had a previous stroke or TIA are at high risk and should routinely receive warfarin as secondary prevention unless contra-indicated.

In primary prevention patients over the age of 75, or between 65–75 with additional independent risk factors such as diabetes, hypertension, or heart failure should receive warfarin. Patients between the age of 65–75 with no additional risk factors, or under 65 with one additional risk factor are at moderate risk of thromboembolism (4% per year) and can be treated with aspirin. Patients under 65 with lone atrial fibrillation have a very low annual incidence of thromboembolism and do not need antithrombotic prophlaxis.

The risk of thromboembolism in patients with chronic atrial fibrillation and paroxysmal atrial fibrillation appears to be similar, independent of the frequency of fibrillation in the paroxysmal group.

Cardioversion should be attempted in all patients with a history of recent onset atrial fibrillation, no structural heart disease, or a correctable precipitating cause. Cardioversion is unlikely to succeed if atrial fibrillation has been present for over 3 months.

The thromboembolic risk from electrical or pharmacological cardioversion is 1–3%. In atrial fibrillation of greater than 48 hours duration patients should be anticoagulated for 3 weeks before cardioversion and continued for at least four weeks afterwards. Following DC cardioversion only 10–30% of cases remain in sinus rythmn at 1 year. Factors associated with this are young age, recent onset AF, structurally normal heart, left atrial size <4.5cm. Antiarrythmic drugs may help sustain sinus rythmn following successful cardioversion though the most appropriate drug and duration of therapy remains controversial.

Drugs that are helpful in restoring sinus rythmn in atrial fibrillation are Class I antiarrythmics such as flecainide and propafenone, Class III such as amiodarone and sotalol and Class IV eg verapamil.

Factors predisposing to the development of atrial fibrillation include ischaemic heart disease, hypertension, rheumatic heart disease, pre-excitation syndromes such as Wolff-Parkinson-White and Lown-Ganong-Levine syndromes, thyrotoxicosis, alcohol, infection esp pneumonia, lung cancer, pulmonary embolism, cardiomyopathy, atrial septal defect, atrial myxoma.

Lip GY et al. The ABC of Atrial Fibrillation
BMJ Publishers 1996

Falk RH. Atrial Fibrillation
NEJM 2001 344; 14: 1067–1078

Question 34

A. false **B.** false **C.** true **D.** true **E.** true

Left venticular hypertrophy (LVH) is the response of the heart to persistent pressure or volume overload. In the Framingham study 16% of men and 19% of women had left venticular hypertrophy. Age, blood pressure, obesity, valvular heart disease and myocardial infarction are all independently associated with left ventricular hypertrophy. There is an increased incidence of cardiovascular disease, stroke and all cause mortality in these subjects. A consequence of LVH is a reduction in coronary artery blood flow which can precipitate ischaemia due to an inability of the coronary microvasculature to vasodilate normally. Recent trials have shown antihypertensives, in particular ACE inhibitors, to reduce and possibly completely reverse left venticular hypertrophy. In the SOLVD study a retrospective analysis showed ACE inhibitors to reduce morbidity, mortality, and the need for hospital admission in hypertensive patients with impaired left ventricular function.

Causes of left ventricular hypertrophy include:

Pressure overload – hypertension, aortic stenosis, co-arctation of the aorta
Volume overload – endurance exercise, mitral regurgitation, aortic regurgitation, pregnancy, obesity
Thyrotoxicosis
Hypertrophic obstructive cardiomyopathy
Cardiac transplantation of undersized hearts
Reactive hypertrophy following cardiac arrest

M-mode echocardiography is most widely used to measure left ventricular mass but is operator dependant and may give erroneous results in distorted ventricles. Two and three dimensional echocardiograpny are more precise but are also more costly and time consuming. MRI provides highly accurate left venticular mass measurements but at present is only used as a research tool.

Lovell B et al. Left ventricular hypertrophy: pathogenesis, detection and prognosis. Circulation 2000 102(4): 470–9

Question 35

A. true **B.** false **C.** false **D.** true **E.** true

Coronary artery bypass grafting (CABG) is a relatively safe procedure with mortality of less than 1% when undertaken by an experienced operator on a subject with normal left ventricular function and no comorbidity. Intraoperative and postoperative mortality increases with degree of ventricular dysfunction, age, comorbidity, and surgical inexperience. Occlusion of vein grafts is seen in 10–20% in the first postoperative year and subsequently in 2% per year for the next 5–7 years. Long-term patency rates are higher following internal mammary artery implantation than saphenous vein grafting. Angina is abolished or greatly reduced in over 90% of subjects following revascularisation though the incidence of myocardial infarction does not appear to be affected. Following revascularisation mortality is reduced in patients who had three vessel or left main coronary artery disease. There have been several trials comparing percutaneous transluminal coronary angioplasty (PTCA) with CABG in patients with multivessel disease. Patients with single or two vessel disease, normal LV function and amenable lesions are recommended to undergo PTCA first though the recurrence of angina and stenosis with the need for subsequent revascularisation approaches 50%. Patients with two or three vessel disease and impaired left venticular function or diabetes should be considered for CABG. Complications following CABG include myocardial infarction, stroke, respiratory impairment and neuropsychiatric abnormalities. Myocardial infarctions occurs in 10–20% of cases and whilst commonly small are the leading cause of peri-operative mortality. Strokes occur in approximately 1% of cases. Neuropsychiatric abnormalities including difficulty in concentration, memory loss, personality change, and depression can occur as a result of cardiopulmonary bypass. The efffects are most marked in the elderly and whilst generally transient can occasionally be permanent.

Julian DG. Disease of the Heart. 2nd Ed. 1998 WB Saunders, Philadelphia.

Question 36

A. false **B.** true **C.** true **D.** false **E.** true

A raised white cell count is found in over 90% of cases of bacterial meningitis with a count of >100wbc/μl being typical with neutrophils predominating in over 80% of cases. Low or undetectable CSF glucose is usual with a simultaneous CSF/plasma ratio of <0.31. However in early bacterial meningitis, partially treated meningitis, and infection with listeria monocytogenes, lymphocytes may predominate making differentiation difficult from viral, tuberculoid, and fungal meningitis.

Low CSF glucose also occurs in tuberculoid meningitis, syphilis, parasitic meningitis, fungal meningitis, herpes simplex encephalitis, carcinomatous meningitis, cerebral vasculitis, aseptic meningitis, and post subarachnoid haemorrhage. Viral infections are associated with a normal CSF glucose.

Acute infective polyradiculopathy causes a raised CSF protein, normal glucose and normal cell count.

Causes of raised CSF protein include meningitis, encephalitis, multiple sclerosis, syphilis, Guillain-Barré, spinal cord block, diabetes, hypothyroidism, subarachnoid haemorrhage, cerebral infarction, intracranial tumour, neurocysticercosis.

Mollarets meningitis (benign recurrent aseptic meningitis) causes a lymphocyte pleocytosis, mildly elevated CSF protein and low to normal CSF glucose. Spontaneous recovery usually occurs within a few days.

Crook DWM, Phuapradit P, Warrell DA. Bacterial meningitis
Oxford Textbook of Medicine. Oxford University Press.

Question 37

A. true **B.** false **C.** false **D.** false **E.** true

Benign intracranial hypertension or pseudotumor cerebri is the syndrome of raised intracranial pressure in the absence of a space occupying lesion or hydrocephalus. It has an incidence of 1:100,00 in the general population rising to 19:100,000 in obese young women. It is very rarely familial. Symptoms and signs are those of raised intracranial pressure with preservation of cerebral function and the absence of focal neurology or epilepsy. Presentation is typically with a headache of weeks to months duration, worse on waking, straining or coughing in association with visual loss. Papilloedema is universal, usually moderate and occasionally unilateral. Visual obscurations, scotoma or persistent blurring occurs in 30–70% of cases. Horizontal diplopia may occur due to a false localizing VI nerve palsy which can be bilateral.

Most cases are idiopathic though there is an association with dural sinus thrombosis, drugs (esp. tetracycline, retinoids, nalidixic acid, nitrofurantoin, lithium, corticosteroids), vitamin A deficiency, and pregnancy. Empty sella syndrome occurs in 4% of cases.

The pathogenesis is unknown but there is thought to be a defect of CSF absorption by the arachnoid villi in the superior sagittal sinus.

The diagnosis is made by demonstrating an elevated CSF pressure of >200mm CSF on lumbar puncture following exclusion of a space occupying lesion or hydrocephalus. The CSF composition is normal. It should be noted that simple obesity can cause an elevated CSF pressure of up to 250mm CSF so the clinical context needs to be considered. Dural sinus thrombosis should be excluded by digital subtraction or MR angiography.

Treatment options include weight loss, thiazide diuretics or acetazolamide, corticosteroids, therapeutic lumbar puncture or in resistant cases surgical lumboperitoneal shunting or optic nerve decompression. Permanent visual loss occurs in up to 50% of cases and is severe in 10%.

Lawton NF. Benign intracranial hypertension
Oxford Textbook of Medicine. Oxford University Press.

Question 38

A. true **B.** false **C.** false **D.** true **E.** false

Anatomical variations of the arterial origin of the posterior cerebral arteries from the basilar artery or internal carotid artery means atypical or incomplete stroke syndromes are commonly produced. Two main syndromes are commonly observed with involvement of either the midbrain and thalamus, or cortical, temporal and occipital lobes.

Occlusion of the proximal left cerebral artery causes midbrain infarction with involvement of the subthalamic nuclei, thalamus and cerebral peduncles. This can give rise to ataxic hemiplegia, hemiballismus, and loss of upward gaze. Extensive infarction in the midbrain causes coma, bilateral pyramidal signs, and decerebrate rigidity.

Weber's syndrome of a 3rd nerve palsy and contralateral hemiplegia, or Claude's syndrome of a 3rd nerve palsy and contralateral ataxia may occur. Distal obstruction of the posterior cerebral artery gives rise to contralateral quadrantic or homonymous hemianopia. When the dominant hemisphere is affected the patient may develop alexia (disturbance of reading) without agraphia, and visual agnosia for faces, objects, and colours. Bilateral infarction of the distal posterior cerebral arteries causes cortical blindness.

The clinical findings in left posterior cerebral artery infarction include right homonymous hemianopia, right visual spatial hemineglect, difficulty naming visual stimuli, and alexia with spared writing along with the Dejerine-Roussy syndrome of altered sensation where occlusion of the thalamic branches arising from the posterior cerebral artery causes hemiparesis with choreiform movements, ataxia and hyperesthesia often with severe paroxysmal pain.

Decerebrate responses are frequent in patients with extensive infarction, and pontine haemorrhage. Wernickes aphasia arises from involvement of the posterior part of the dominant cerebral hemisphere supplied by branches of the middle cerebral artery.

Hohr JP, Pessin MS. Posterior Cerebral Artery Disease
Stroke. 3rd Edition. 1998 Churchill Livingstone. Pennsylvania.

Question 39

A. true **B.** true **C.** false **D.** false **E.** true

Neurological complications are common in rheumatoid arthritis and related to nerve compression, disuse atrophy, steroid myopathy or vasculitis. They include:

Inflammatory myositis
Peripheral neuropathy (predominantly sensory)
Mononeuritis multiplex
Nerve compression syndromes (esp carpal tunnel syndrome and ulnar nerve lesions)
Atlantoaxial or subaxial subluxation which is commoner in women on steroids. This gives rise to a cervical myelopathy and can range from brisk reflexes to a para or tetra-paresis
C2 (occipital) root pain

Other cause of mononeuritis multiplex include diabetes mellitus, sarcoidosis, vasculitis (eg. Churg-Strauss syndrome, Wegener's granulomatosis, polyarteritis nodosa) paraneoplastic syndromes, HIV infection, leprosy, serum sickness reactions, and primary hyperoxaluria.

Harrison MJG Neurological Complications of Systemic Diseases.
Oxford Textbook of Medicine. Oxford University Press.

Question 40

A. true **B.** true **C.** true **D.** true **E.** true

Psychiatric disorders of eating include anorexia nervosa, bulimia nervosa, psychogenic vomiting and obesity.

Clinical features of Anorexia Nervosa:

Excessive concern with shape and weight; morbid fear of fatness

Distorted body image

Over representation of cases from upper socio-economic groups

Pursuit of thinness with consequent low body weight through dieting, avoidance of carbohydrate, self-induced vomiting, compulsive exercising, purging, obsessional, symptoms related to eating.

Preoccupation with food (can involve binge-eating)

Amenorrhoea

Low mood, often frank clinical depression; also mood lability, irritability and anxiety.

Lack of sexual interest

Consequences of starvation include emaciation, constipation, low blood pressure, bradycardia, sensitivity to cold, hypothermia, consequences of laxative and diuretic abuse, and vomiting, alkalosis, hypokalaemia, family history of psychiatric illness.

Fine, downy lanugo hair on back, arms and side of face.

Clinical features of Bulimia nervosa

Usually older than anorexia nervosa patients

Broader class distribution

Depressive and anxiety symptoms more marked than in anorexia nervosa

Excessive concern with shape and weight

Binge eating

Behaviour to prevent weight gain (dietary restraint, self-induced vomiting, compulsive exercising purging)

Consequent normal body weight

Consequences of potassium depletion (weakness, oedema, cardiac arrhythmias, renal impairment)

Other consequences of repeated vomiting include swollen parotid glands, pitted teeth

Family history of psychiatric illness

Psychiatry and Medicine. In Gelder M, Mayou R, Geddes J, eds. Psychiatry, Oxford: Oxford University Press, 1999.

Question 41

A. true **B.** false **C.** true **D.** true **E.** true

Features of hyperventilation:

Rapid, shallow breathing, with a subjective experience of breathlessness; generally not an experience of overbreathing.
Tachycardia
Dizziness or light-headedness
Tinnitus
Headache
Precordial discomfort
Weakness
Faintness
Numbness and tingling in hands and feet, or around the mouth
Paraesthesia of the extremities
Carpopedal spasm
Visual disturbances; difficulty in focusing vision, blurred vision.

Overbreathing lowers arterial pCO_2 and causes a respiratory alkalosis. This reduces the ionised calcium, causing functional hypocalcaemia, which leads to the paraesthesia, carpopedal spasm and even fitting. Asking the patient to overbreathe in outpatients / casualty can often reproduce the symptoms and is the best test.

Psychiatry and Medicine. In Gelder M, Mayou R, Geddes J, eds. Psychiatry, Oxford: Oxford University Press, 1999.

Question 42

A. true **B.** true **C.** false **D.** true **E.** true

The CAGE questions

Have you ever felt you needed to Cut down on your drinking?
Do you feel Angry when people question you about your drinking?
Do you feel Guilty about your drinking?
Do you have an Eye opener? (early morning drinking)

are probably familiar to most medical students. Monday morning absenteeism is another important sign of alcoholism.

Alcoholics rarely actually get drunk – they maintain an even drinking pattern during waking hours to maintain their serum level of alcohol and avoid the 'shakes'; their tolerance to alcohol is higher as evidenced by their ability to consume one or more bottles of vodka per day, typical of alcohol dependence.

Alcohol advisory services advocate complete abstinence. Even small amounts of alcohol re-establish the previous drinking patterns. Alcohol dependence often leads to failed relationships, unemployment and social withdrawal as drinking takes over from other activities.

Confusion in the alcoholic patient: a differential diagnosis

Acute intoxication
Delerium tremens (48–72 hrs post-withdrawal)
Hypoglycaemia (6–36 h post binge)
Head injury leading to subdural haematoma
Post ictal
Wernicke – Korsakoff syndrome
Ketoacidosis or lactic acidosis
Hepatic encephalopathy
Sepsis (eg Klebsiella pneumonia, aspiration pneumonia)
Unusual neurological syndromes eg central pontine myelinolysis

Mark Ashworth and Claire Gerada. ABC of mental health: Addiction and dependence II: Alcohol. BMJ 1997 315: 358–360.

Question 43

A. true **B.** true **C.** false **D.** false **E.** false

Anorexia and bulimia have been discussed in Paper 1 Question 40. Frontal lobe neoplasia causes disinhibition. A flat, blunted affect is one of the negative symptoms of schizophrenia. The others include:

Underactivity
Lack of motivation
Social withdrawal
Emotional apathy

Mood disorder
Blunting of affect
Incongruity; when emotions do appear they are often inappropriate
Depression

Thought disorder
Abnormality of the amount and speed of thought
Abnormality of the ways in which thoughts are linked
Delusions; often persecutory
Overvalued ideas
Obsessional/compulsive symptoms

Hallucinations, usually auditory
Impaired insight

Potentially misleading presentations of depression:

Anorexia, weight loss
Fatigue
Constipation
Loss of libido
Amenorrhea
Sleep disturbance

Schizophrenia and related disorders. In Gelder M, Mayou R, Geddes J, eds. Psychiatry, Oxford: Oxford University Press, 1999.

Question 44

A. true **B**. false **C**. true **D**. true **E**. true

Bronchiectasis describes abnormal chronic dilatation of the bronchi characterized clinically by cough, excessive sputum production, recurrent chest infections, and in severe cases finger clubbing and interstitial fibrosis. 10% of affected individuals suffer from some form of immune deficiency.

Treatment consists of postural drainage, prompt antibiotic treatment of infective exacerbations, bronchodilators, steroids. Surgery is reserved for the treatment of localized disease or complications such as massive haemoptysis.

Prophylactic treatment with oral or nebulised antibiotics 2–3/week may be useful in patients with frequent recurrent infections though resistance can be a problem.

Causes of bronchiectasis include

Infections:	Tuberculosis, Measles, Whooping cough, Mycoplasma pneumonia, Adenovirus
Immune deficiency:	Immunoglobulin deficiency (primary and secondary) Complement deficiency, Chronic granulomatous disorder, Chediak-Higashi syndrome
Hyperimmune states:	Post lung transplant, Allergic bronchopulmonary aspergillosis
Mucociliary clearance defects:	Ciliary dyskinesia (Kartageners syndrome when associated with dextrocardia and situs inversus), Youngs syndrome, Cystic fibrosis
Bronchial obstruction:	Foreign body inhalation, Lymph node, Malignancy

Others: Aspiration pneumonia
Pulmonary fibrosis
Alpha-1-antitrypsin deficiency
Yellow nail syndrome

CXR changes include

Tramline shadows
Cystic lesions (may be fluid filled)
Volume loss with crowding of vessels
Areas of atelectasis
Fibrosis

Stockley RA. Bronchiectasis
Oxford Textbook of Medicine. Oxford University Press.

Question 45

A. false **B.** false **C.** false **D.** false **E.** false

This question is testing your ability to recognize and treat appropriately acute severe asthma. The British Thoracic Society produced guidelines on the management of asthma in 1990 which were subsequently updated in 1997 and which you are well advised to study. (See reference)

Symptoms of severe asthma include

the inability to talk in sentences
respiratory rate >25/min
tachycardia >110/min
PEFR < 50% of predicted
Additional life threatening features include silent chest, poor respiratory effort, low respiratory rate, confusion, exhaustion, bradycardia, hypotension, PEFR < 30% predicted

All patients presenting with an acute asthma attack should have arterial blood gas analysis. Pulse oximetry is not an acceptable alternative. A normal/elevated pCO_2 and normal/low pH are indicators of life-threatening asthma and as such they need to be assessed in all patients that require hospital admission. Intravenous steroids have a slow onset of action, (4–6hrs), and whilst they should be given early as part of the emergency management of asthma, they do not effect the initial course of the attack. High flow oxygen should be given as carbon dioxide retention is rarely a concern.

British Thoracic Society (1997). British guidelines on asthma management
Thorax 1997; 52: S1–24

Busse WW, Lemanske RF. Asthma
NEJM 2001 344; 5: 350–362

Question 46

A. false **B.** false **C.** false **D.** false **E.** true

Extrinsic allergic alveolitis (EAA) or hypersensitivity pneumonitis is diffuse pulmonary inflammation in response to inhaled organic dusts. Farmers lung is the most common cause secondary to aspergillus fumigatus. There are a wide range of other agents, most commonly micro-organisms, that have been reported to cause EAA. In its acute form a sensitized subject develops a flu-like illness with cough, dyspnoea and rarely wheeze 3–9 hours following exposure. Spontaneous recovery usually starts within 24 hours of removal from the source. Clinically the patient is febrile, has basal crepitations, and may have alveolar shadowing on CXR. Treatment with steroids will accelerate remission. The chronic form of the disease usually develops in response to low-level antigenic exposure over a number of years such as in Bird fanciers lung. The onset is insidious with gradually progressive pulmonary fibrosis that ultimately leads to pulmonary hypertension and cor pulmonale. Smoking appears to protect against the development of EAA.

Originally EAA was thought to develop from immune-complex deposition however the evidence for this is actually quite weak. Fluid obtained at bronchoalveolar lavage in patients with a current attack reveals a consistent acute T-lymphocyte response which supports the recent change in consensus that the immune pathology is a T-cell mediated delayed-type hypersensitivity response with granuloma formation. (This is in disagreement with the college answer in stem b). Peripheral eosinophilia does not occur. Precipitating antibodies are present in the serum but indicate antigenic exposure rather than disease.

Hendrick DJ. Extrinsic Allergic Alveolitis
Ledingham JGG, Warrell DA. Concise Oxford Textbook of Medicine 2000
Oxford University Press. Oxford.

Question 47

A. false **B.** false **C.** false **D.** false **E.** true

Siderosis (iron) and stannosis (tin) are benign pneumoconioses with CXR changes due to radio-opaque material taken up by macrophages. The changes regress completely when exposure ceases and pulmonary fibrosis does not develop.

Byssinosis (cotton) is airway hyper-responsiveness to cotton dust. An asthma-like picture develops in cotton mill workers following long-term exposure but this does not progress to chronic lung disease.

Aspergillus spores are ubiquitous in the environment and are readily inhaled but only rarely cause disease. Allergic bronchopulmonary aspergillosis results from aspergillus growing in the bronchi causing an eosinophilic reaction. It is the hyphae that stimulate an immune response which can lead to the development of proximal bronchiectasis and predominantly upper lobe fibrosis. Aspergillomas may develop in old lung cavities most commonly secondary to previous tuberculosis, and rarely in immunocompromised hosts invasive aspergillosis may develop which has a poor prognosis.

Causes of pulmonary fibrosis include

RHEUMATOLOGICAL AND CONNECTIVE TISSUE DISORDERS
Scleroderma
SLE
Rheumatoid arthritis
Ankylosing spondylitis
Polymyositis

VASCULITIDES
Wegener's granulomatosis
Churg-Strauss syndrome
Microscopic polyangiitis

GRANULOMATOUS DISEASE
Sarcoidosis
Histiocytosis X
Tuberculosis

DRUGS
Amiodarone
Nitrofurantoin
Cytotoxic agents

MALIGNANCY
Lymphoma
Lymphangitis carcinomatosa

PNEUMOCONIOSIS
Asbestos
Coal
Silica
Beryllium

MISCELLANEOUS
Extrinsic allergic alveolitis
Alveolar proteinosis
Lymphangioleiomyomatosis
Tuberous sclerosis
Neurofibromatosis

Woodcock AA, Du Bois RM. Parenchymal Lung Disease
Ledingham JGG, Warrell DA. Concise Oxford Textbook of Medicine 2000
Oxford University Press. Oxford.

Question 48

A. true **B.** true **C.** false **D.** true **E.** true

Coeliac disease is an inflammatory disease of the upper small intestine resulting from gluten ingestion in genetically susceptible individuals. The inflammation results in malabsorption of several nutrients. These can cause general malaise including mouth ulcers as well as specific problems such as osteomalacia from calcium malabsorption and reduction in proteins such as albumin and serum ferritin.

The endomysial antibody test is the most accurate, and most widely available serological test, with some authors claiming close to 100% sensitivity and specificity. Serum anti-tissue transglutaminase shows some promise.

Histological evidence of gluten sensitive enteropathy is regarded as the gold standard for diagnosis of coeliac disease, with subtotal villous atrophy, an increase in intraepithelial lymphocytes and plasma cells.

Symptoms and signs of coeliac disease:

Infancy (<2 years):
Diarrhoea
Abdominal distension
Failure to thrive
Anorexia and vomiting

Childhood
Diarrhoea and constipation
Anaemia (usually iron-deficiency)
Loss of appetite (short stature, osteoporosis)

Adulthood
Diarrhoea or constipation
Anaemia
Aphthous ulcers, sore tongue and mouth
Dyspepsia, abdominal pain, bloating and weight loss
Fatigue, anxiety and depression
Bone pain (osteomalacia and/or osteoporosis)
Splenic atrophy

James MW, Scott BB. Endomysial antibodies in the diagnosis and management of coeliac disease. Postgrad Med J 2000; 76: 466–468.

Schuppan D. Current concepts of Coeliac Disease Pathogenesis. Gastroenterology 2000; 119: 234–242

Question 49

A. true **B.** true **C.** true **D.** true **E.** false

Cholesterol stones are associated with:

Ethnicity
Older age
Female gender
Obesity
Diet
Drugs (eg. Oral contraceptive pill, clofibrate)
Gastrointestinal disease (Crohns disease)

Bile pigment stones are associated with: increasing with age, cirrhosis, chronic bile duct obstruction, chronic haemolysis, (eg. heart valve-induced, malaria). The incidence is equal in males and females.

Pyoderma gangrenosum is associated with both Crohn's disease and ulcerative colitis. It is particularly troublesome when it forms peri-stomally. Gallstones are associated with Crohn's disease; patients with short-bowel syndrome almost invariably have stones, and up to 50% of these are symptomatic.

Oxaluria and oxalate stones are particularly common in ileal disease and with steatorrhoea of any cause. The mechanism is linked to the binding of calcium to unabsorbed fat, leaving oxalate free to be absorbed in the colon.

Crohn's disease is a cause of amyloid due to its chronic inflammatory nature; it does occur in ulcerative colitis but it is much less common. Dermatitis herpetiformis is associated with Coeliac disease not Crohn's disease. It may present as a separate entitity with a gluten sensitive rash without the enteropathy normally associated with coeliac disease. Any patient presenting with Dermatitis herpetiformis de novo should have an endoscopy and small bowel biopsy.

Amyloid:

AL: primary, light chains are deposited in tissues, eg. Waldenstom's, myeloma

AA: reactive or secondary, due to acute phase proteins in chronic inflammation. Eg. Rheumatoid arthritis, bronchiectasis, familial Mediterranean fever, low grade malignancy (Crohn's less common)

Effects of AA:

Kidney – nephritic syndrome can lead to chronic renal failure
Liver, Spleen – hepatosplenomegaly
Adrenal glands – hypoadrenalism
Gut – diarrhoea, malabsorption
Does not affect the heart

AL gives effects of AA and:

Large tongue
Telangiectasia from ruptured skin capillaries
Palpable peripheral neuropathy
Heart: restrictive cardiomyopathy (do NOT give digoxin!)
Coagulopathy

Beta-2 microglobulin:

In haemodialysis
A constituent of class I HLA
Accumulates in brain and heart in old age

Familial Mediterranean Fever:

Can cause various familial amyloid polyneuropathic disorders.

Jewell DP. Crohns disease. In Weatherall DJ, Ledingham JGG, Warrell DA, eds. Oxford Textbook of Medicine, Oxford: Oxford University Press, 1996.

Question 50

A. true **B.** true **C.** false **D.** true **E.** false

Below are the diagnostic (Rome) criteria for irritable bowel syndrome; generally these are signs of functional bowel disorder, although of course one still must be careful not to miss organic disease.

A history of at least 12 weeks, which need not be consecutive, in the preceding 12 months of abdominal discomfort or pain that has two out of three of the following features:

1. relieved with defecation; and/or
2. onset associated with a change in frequency of stool; and/or
3. onset associated with a change in form (appearance) of stool.

Although not formally part of the criteria, the symptoms below cumulatively support the diagnosis of irritable bowel syndrome:

1. abnormal stool frequency (for research purposes abnormal may be defined as greater that 3 bowel movements per day and less than 3 bowel movements per week);
2. abnormal stool form (lumpy/hard or loose/watery stool);
3. abnormal stool passage (straining, urgency, or feeling of incomplete evacuation);
5. passage of mucus;
6. bloating or feeling of abdominal distension.

Patients with warning signs such as weight loss, abdominal distension, pain waking them up at night, or waking up at night to defaecate are more likely to have organic disease and must be investigated accordingly.

Camilleri M. Management of the Irritable Bowel Syndrome
Gastroenterology 2001 120: 652–668
Horwitz BJ, Fisher RS. The Irritable Bowel Syndrome
NEJM 2001 344; 24: 1846–1850

Question 51

A. false **B.** true **C.** true **D.** false **E.** true

Gastro-oesophageal reflux disease (GORD) occurs when acid gastric contents reflux into the oesophagus, and is also associated with impaired clearance. It is not synonymous with hiatus hernia or ulceration of the oesophagus; in fact oesophageal ulceration only occurs in around 5% of cases. (Therefore the normal endoscopy does not exclude the diagnosis). Delayed gastric emptying is common, although there is little evidence that prokinetic drugs are useful in GORD. Symptoms will not resolve after H pylori eradication, although typically the symptoms resolve while the proton pump inhibitor is given during the eradication period. Up to 20% of GORD patients have Barretts oesophagus, which is the development of metaplastic columnar epithelium in the distal lining of the oesophagus. Although the management of Barretts proves to be controversial its significance does not: it is associated with dysplasia and/or frank malignancy hence the periodic surveillance of patients with Barretts in endoscopy units.

McDougall NI, Johnston BT, Kee F et al. Natural history of reflux oesophagitis: a 10 year follow up of its effect on patient symptomatology and quality of life. Gut 1996; 38: 481–6

Chiba N, Hunt RH. Gastroesophageal reflux disease. McDonald J, Feagan B, Burroughs A, eds. Evidence Based Gastroenterology and Hepatology, London: BMJ Books, 1999.

Question 52

A. true **B.** false **C.** false **D.** true **E.** false

ACTH can be produced from many tumours, especially small cell lung carcinoma, but also pancreatic islet tumours, bronchial carcinoid, thyroid medullary carcinoma, phaeochromocytoma and prostatic carcinoma. Small cell lung carcinoma can also produce ADH, CRH and GHRH.

ACTH production tends to be in rapidly growing tumours, so symptoms of Cushing's syndrome, particularly chronic ones, tend to be blunted. Hypokalaemia, muscle weakness, weight loss and glucose intolerance tend to predominate. Hypokalaemia, hypochloraemia and resulting metabolic alkalosis are particularly marked in ectopic ACTH production, accounting for the elevated bicarbonate concentration. If the ACTH is from a small cell carcinoma then the clinical presentation more commonly resembles Addison's rather than Cushing's syndrome and patients are commonly pigmented in addition to the signs described above. Patients with benign tumours, such as bronchial carcinoids that produce ACTH, present with the typical features of Cushing's syndrome. There are no reports of calcium being affected by ACTH production.

The ACTH concentration is typically high in the above tumours, and as the production is ectopic and autonomous it is not affected by dexamethasone administration. This is the principal way to determine the difference between ectopic ACTH related Cushing's syndrome and the Cushing's syndrome of pituitary origin.

Edwards CRW. Adrenocortical diseases. In Weatherall DJ, Ledingham JGG, Warrell DA, eds. Oxford Textbook of Medicine, Oxford: Oxford University Press, 1996.

Question 53

A. false **B.** true **C.** false **D.** true **E.** true

Primary hyperparathyroidism is caused by an increase in circulating concentrations of parathyroid hormone (PTH). It implies hyperfunction of one or more parathyroid glands resulting in raised PTH and hypercalcaemia. It is usually due to a single parathyroid adenoma of the chief cells, or more rarely due to diffuse hyperplasia or multiple adenomata. Carcinoma is very rare.

Primary hyperparathyroidism can resemble rickets in children, due to resorption of metaphyseal bone. Cystic lesions may be found, and the skull resorption may give a mottled, salt and pepper appearance. Other features are due to hypercalcaemia, and are often very vague, including nausea, vomiting, fatigue, constipation and hypotonicity. The hypercalcaemia induces polyuria, leading to dehydration or polydipsia.

Patients may have laboratory values of PTH within the normal ranges that in the presence of hypercalcaemia are inappropriately high, or may have normal calcium levels, but with an inappropriately raised PTH. There are cases where patients with primary hyperparathyroidism are normocalcaemic because of coexistent vitamin D deficiency. Hypomagnesaemia (not hypermagnasaemia) is a recognized though uncommon finding in primary hyperparathyroidism.

Postoperative tetany due to hypocalcaemia is said to be common in patients with diffuse bone disease, and these patients are usually treated with intravenous calcium as well as starting vitamin D.

Acute pancreatitis, although not common is a recognized feature of hypercalcaemia.

Neurological disturbances range from mild behavioural disorders to psychosis, sometimes-reversible dementia, and focal neurological lesions.

Kanis JA. Disorders of Calcium metabolism. In Weatherall DJ, Ledingham JGG, Warrell DA, eds. Oxford Textbook of Medicine, Oxford: Oxford University Press, 1996

Marx SJ. Hyperparathyroid and hypoparathyroid disorders NEJM 2000 343; 25: 1863–1875

Question 54

A. true **B.** false **C.** false **D.** true **E.** false

Papillary thyroid carcinoma is the most common malignant thyroid tumour. It is more common in women (3:1) and is most frequent in the third to fourth decade. They are locally invasive, and occasionally multifocal. The disease ranges from small papillary cancers, found in 6–13% of autopsied American patients to sclerosing, diffuse carcinomas that can infiltrate the whole thyroid.

Papillary carcinoma is relatively benign overall with 10–20 year recurrence rates of about 5% and death rates of 2–5%. In contrast follicular thyroid carcinoma is more aggressive, distant metastases develop in about 20% of patients, and the 5-year mortality rates are about 60%.

Surgery is the preferred method of treatment for papillary carcinoma, with or without radio-iodine (I^{131}) treatment. Whilst radio-iodine is controversial for different stages of the disease it has an established role in residual and in metastatic disease. Different commentators vary in their indications for treatment with radio-iodine.

Rossi RL, Majlis S, Rossi RM. Thyroid cancer. Surgical Clinics of North America 2000 80(2): 571–580

Question 55

A. false **B.** true **C.** true **D.** true **E.** true

Autoimmune Addison's disease may be both sporadic or due to polyglandular autoimmune syndromes. Skin pigmentation is generally seen in sun-exposed areas, recent scars, axillae, nipples, palmar creases, mucous membranes and pressure points. There may be associated vitiligo. Other autoimmune conditions may be related, such as pernicious anaemia and ovarian failure. The combination of hypothyroidism and autoimmune Addison's is known as Schmidt's syndrome.

The patient may present with hypotension and acute circulatory failure, described as an Addisonian crisis. Anorexia and weight loss are early features, which may progress to nausea, vomiting and diarrhoea. Often crises are precipitated by intercurrent infection and stress, such as surgery. Other features of chronic adrenal insufficiency are weakness, easy fatigability, weight loss, muscle cramps, postural hypotension as well as general malaise and the GI side effects above.

Hyponatraemia is present in 90% of cases and hyperkalaemia in 65%. Blood urea and nitrogen concentrations are usually raised; eosinophilia, hypoglycaemia and raised ESR are often present.

Addison's description of the disease was secondary to Tuberculosis. Autoimmune causes are the most frequent accounting for 70% of presentations. Other rare causes:

Metastatic tumour
Lymphoma
Amyloid
Intra-adrenal haemorrhage (Waterhouse-Friederichsen syndrome) following meningococcal septicaemia
Haemochromatosis
Adrenal infarction or infection other than tuberculosis (especially AIDS)
Adrenoleucodystrophy
Adrenomyeloneuropathy
Hereditary adrenocortical unresponsiveness to ACTH
Bilateral adrenalectomy

Edwards CRW. Adrenocortical diseases. In Weatherall DJ, Ledingham JGG, Warrell DA, eds. Oxford Textbook of Medicine, Oxford: Oxford University Press, 1996.

Question 56

A. false **B.** false **C.** false **D.** true **E.** true

Renal tubular acidosis is characterized by an inability to acidify the urine appropriately in response to systemic acidosis. This leads to excess renal chloride resorption to maintain electrical neutrality and the development of a hyperchloraemic hypokalaemic metabolic acidosis with normal anion gap. Distal (type I) renal tubular acidosis typically presents in childhood or early adult life with acute acidosis, hyperventilation, and muscle weakness due to hypokalaemia. 70% of patients have nephrocalcinosis or renal calculi and rickets or osteomalacia may occur as the acidosis prevents resorption of calcium resulting in hypercalciuria and secondary hyperparathyroidism. Type I RTA occurs through a defect in the distal nephron resulting in failure of H^+ secretion and thus bicarbonate resorption. The diagnosis is made by demonstrating a urinary pH >5.5 in the presence of a normal anion gap acidosis. Failure to acidify the urine maximally despite the presence of severe acidosis (plasma HCO_3^- <12mmol/l) distinguishes type I RTA from types II and IV. Type I RTA is most commonly inherited in an autosomal dominant manner though it may occur in association with autoimmune disorders (most commonly

Sjögrens syndrome or primary biliary cirrhosis), or from damage to the renal medulla (eg pyelonephritis, papillary necrosis, medullary sponge kidney, analgesic nephropathy).

Proximal (type II) renal tubular acidosis results from a defect in HCO_3^- secretion in the proximal tubule and is usually associated with other tubular abnormalities such as glycosuria, aminoaciduria, hyperphosphaturia, and uricosuria (Fanconi syndrome). The urine can maximally acidify in the presence of severe acidosis and nephrocalcinosis and renal calculi do not occur. Familial cases are rare and the renal tubular acidosis is usually secondary to generalized proximal tubule damage. Recognized causes include cystinosis, Wilson's disease, hereditary fructose intolerance, multiple myeloma, lead poisoning, outdated tetracycline therapy, hyperparathyroidism, and the nephrotic syndrome. Large quantities of sodium bicarbonate may be necessary for treatment.

Type IV renal tubular acidosis presents with a hyperkalaemic hyperchloraemic normal anion gap acidosis. This is generally in response to hypoaldosteronism either secondary to Addison's disease or due to low renin production as seen in diabetes and chronic tubulointerstitial disease or secondary to NSAID use. Mineralocorticoid should be used for treatment if the acidosis is severe.

Unwin RJ, Capasso G. The Renal Tudular Acidoses
J R Soc Med 2001; 94: 221–225

Question 57

A. false **B.** true **C.** false **D.** false **E.** true

Prostate specific antigen is a serine protease produced by both normal and malignant prostate epithelial cells. It is a very sensitive indicator for prostatic cancer though widespread acceptance of screening remains controversial as there are concerns that small insignificant tumours may be detected along with tumours that have spread outside the capsule and are thus incurable. High values are sensitive and specific for the diagnosis of prostatic cancer but diagnostic confusion remains between benign prostatic hypertrophy and prostate cancer at mildly elevated levels just outside the normal range. Increased specificity for prostatic cancer can be gained from calculating prostate specific antigen density by dividing the serum antigen level by the volume of the gland as determined at transrectal ultrasound.

Causes of a raised PSA include age, acute retention, catheterization, transurethral prostate resection, prostatitis, prostate biopsy, benign prostatic hypertrophy, and prostatic cancer.

Dawson C, Whitfield H. ABC of Urology
BMJ publishing group 1997

Barry MJ, PSA Testing for early diagnosis of prostate cancer. NEJM 2001, 344: 1373-1377

Question 58

A. true **B.** false **C.** false **D.** true **E.** false

Contrast nephropathy is one of the commonest causes of drug-induced acute renal failure. Renal failure develops within 2 days of the injection with a peak in creatinine 2–4 days later with most cases recovering within a week. Occasionally dialysis may be required particularly if the baseline creatinine was above 300mmol/l though the development of endstage renal failure is rare. The major risk factors for the development of contrast nephropathy are pre-existing renal failure (Creatinine>140mmol/l), diabetes mellitus, dehydration, solitary kidney, multiple myeloma, and excessive contrast volume. Non-ionic low osmolality contrast medium reduces the incidence of renal toxicity in high risk groups but does not abolish it. Previous studies with prophylactic treatment such as with mannitol, frusemide, or dopamine has not been shown to be of benefit however in a recent study prophylactic oral administration of the antioxidant acetylcysteine, along with hydration, prevented the reduction in renal function induced by iopromide, a nonionic, low-osmolality contrast agent, in patients with chronic renal insufficiency.

Moreau JF, Helenon O, Kinkel K et al. Conventional Uroradiology and Contrast Media

Davidson AM et al. Oxford Text Book of Clinical Nephrology 2nd Ed. 1998

Tepel M et al. Prevention of Radiographic contrast agent induced reductions in renal function by acetylcysteine. NEJM 2000 343; 3: 180–184
Editorial: p211

Question 59

A. false **B.** true **C.** true **D.** false **E.** true

The glomerulonephritides can only present in one of five different ways with either persistent proteinuria, microscopic haematuria, nephrotic syndrome, acute nephritic syndrome, or renal failure.

The acute nephritic syndrome is the combination of acute onset macroscopic haematuria and proteinuria commonly associated with oliguria, hypertension, pulmonary congestion and non-pitting oedema. In contrast to the nephrotic syndrome plasma albumin concentration is maintained. The most common causes are mesangiocapillary glomerulonephritis, IgA nephropathy, post-streptococcal glomerulonephritis, and diffuse proliferative or rapidly progressive glomerulonephritis secondary to Henoch-Schönlein purpura, SLE, or one of the vasculitides.

Membranous nephropathy presents with proteinuria and the nephrotic syndrome. Microscopic haematuria occurs in up to 20% of cases though macroscopic haematuria does not occur. It is commonly idiopathic though 25% of cases are secondary to drugs, malignancy, SLE or chronic hepatitis B infection. 10% of patients on gold or penicillamine develop membranous nephropathy which may persist for up to two years following cessation of treatment though rarely progresses to endstage renal failure. Recent studies have shown 90% of patients with all cause membranous nephropathy to have functioning kidneys after 5 years of follow up. Renal vein thrombosis must be considered in any patient with a sudden deterioration in renal function. Treatment is with steroids +/– chlorambucil though the risks of immunosuppressive therapy must be weighed against the relatively good prognosis the disease carries.

Amyloid nephropathy occurs in nearly all patients with AA (reactive) amyloidosis and at least 50% of AL amyloidosis. Amyloid is initially deposited in the glomeruli and subsequently in the tubules and interstitium. Clinical presentation is most commonly with nephrotic syndrome though occasionally renal tubular acidosis, the Fanconi syndrome or diabetes insipidus may occur. Management is supportive and patients progressing to endstage renal failure may require dialysis or transplantation. Patients on long-term dialysis may develop B2-microglobulin amyloidosis where the amyloid is deposited in joints, tendons, and bones.

Cameron JS. Common Clinical Presentations and Symptoms in Renal Disorders

Ledingham JGG, Warrell DA (Eds). Concise Oxford textbook of Medicine. 2000 Oxford University Press, Oxford

Question 60

A. true **B.** false **C.** false **D.** false **E.** true

Urethritis in men is termed gonococcal or non-gonococcal. 40% of cases of non-gonococcal urethritis are due to infection with Chlamydia trachomatis with the majority of the rest probably due to the fastidious organisms Ureaplasma urealyticum, mycoplasma hominis, and mycoplasma genitalium. Clinically NGU can be indistinguishable from gonococcal urethritis with urethral itching, pain, and a purulent discharge though up to 1/3rd of males with NGU are asymptomatic. Doxycycline is the antimicrobial of choice though recently a single dose of Azithromycin has been proven to be equally effective and may improve patient compliance. NGU has been documented in up to 70% of cases of non-diarrhoeal Reiters syndrome.

Reiters syndrome is the triad of reactive arthritis, conjunctivitis, and non-gonococcal urethritis though a similar syndrome can also be triggered by enteric infection, typically due to Shigella, Salmonella, Campylobacter, or Yersinia. 75% of patients are positive for HLA B27. Clinical findings include asymmetrical polyarthritis, dactylitis, tendinitis and fascitis, conjunctivitis, uveitis, orogenital ulceration, circinate balanitis, keratoderma blenorrhagica (hyperkeratotic vesicular rash over the palms and soles), onycholysis, aortic regurgitation, and pulmonary infiltrates.

Burstein GR et al. Non-gonococcal urethritis a new paradigm. Clinical Infectious Diseases 1999; 28 Suppl: S66–73

Paper 2 Answers

Question 1

A. false **B.** true **C.** true **D.** true **E.** false

Disorders where it is only necessary to carry one abnormal allele in order for an individual to be affected are said to be dominant. In autosomal dominant disorders the abnormal gene is carried on a non- sex chromosome; in X linked disorders, the gene is carried on the X chromosome.

In recessive inheritance, an individual is only affected if he or she does not carry a normal allele at all. For autosomal recessive inheritance, affected individuals will be homozygous for the abnormal allele and both of the parents will be heterozygotes. In X-linked recessive disorders, males homozygous for the abnormal allele will be affected, whereas heterozygous females will be unaffected. All the daughters of an affected male are carriers and all the sons are normal (because a male passes his X chromosome to his daughters and his Y chromosome to his sons). Half of the sons of a carrier female are affected (because they have no compensatory X chromosome) and half of the daughters are carriers.

X linked recessive inheritance:

Carrier Male:	normal female & mother all sons normal all daughters carriers
Carrier Females	normal male & father 50% sons affected, 50% normal 50% daughters carriers, 50% normal

X linked recessive disorders usually manifest in males and females pass on the gene. A female will have the disease if they inherit two affected X chromosomes e.g. in G-6-PD deficiency

Examples:

Haemophilias A & B
Duchenne muscular dystrophy / Beckers dystrophy
Alports syndrome
Lesch Nyhan syndrome
Nephrogenic diabetes insipidus

Testicular feminization syndrome
G-6-PD deficiency
Kennedy syndrome
Ehlers Danlos syndrome (type IX)
Agammaglobulinaemia
Lymphoproliferative syndrome
Wiskott Aldrich syndrome / Emery Dreifuss muscular dystrophy
Inherited idiopathic X linked dystonia

Pembrey ME. Genetic factors in disease
Oxford Textbook of Medicine. Oxford University Press.

Question 2

A. true **B.** false **C.** true **D.** true **E.** true

Some autosomal dominant traits:

Achondroplasia
Acute intermittent porphyria
Adult polycystic kidney disease
Alzheimers disease (some forms)
Epidermolysis bullosa (some forms)
Facioscapulohumeral dystrophy
Familial hypercholesterolaemia
Huntington's chorea
Malignant hyperpyrexia
Myotonic dystrophy
Neurofibromatosis
Noonan's syndrome
Osteogenesis imperfecta
Polyposis coli
Tuberous sclerosis
von Hippel Lindau disease

Autosomal dominant disorders affect both males and females and can be traced through many generations of a family. Affected people are heterozygous for the abnormal allele and pass the gene for the disease to 50% of their offering. If a family member does not have the disease they do not pass it on. Estimation of risk depends on multiple factors:

1. age – some disorders do not manifest themselves until well into adult life e.g. Huntington's chorea / myotonic dystrophy
2. severity of the disorder varies within affected individuals e.g. a parent with tuberous sclerosis with only skin manifestations may have an affected child with infantile spasms and severe mental retardation

3. the disorder may arise out of a new mutation
4. some disorders show a lack of penetrance
5. non genetic factors may play a role e.g. cholesterol intake in hypercholesterolaemia and drugs in porphyria

Kingston HM. ABC of Clinical Genetics
British Medical Association. BMA publishing

Question 3

A. false **B.** true **C.** true **D.** false **E.** true

The polymerase chain reaction involves making copies of a target sequence of DNA (DNA amplification). Therefore the original sequence of DNA that you are studying must already be known. Amplification occurs by using a pair of oligonucleotide primers each complimentary to one end of the DNA target sequence. These are extended towards each other by a thermostable DNA polymerase in a reaction of three steps:

1. Denaturation (e.g. at 95°C) where the DNA to be amplified is heated to produce two strands
2. Annealing: DNA is cooled (e.g. to 55°C) and the two chosen oligonucleotide primers that flank the region of interest bind (anneal) or hybridise to their respective strands

3.) Synthesis: a polymerisation step (e.g. at 72°C) occurs where the primers initiate the synthesis of two new strands of DNA by a thermostable polymerase e.g. Taq polymerase. A thermostable polymerase is used as it will survive the first part of the cycle at 95°C.

Repeating this cycle around 30 times can amplify a single copy of a DNA sequence 100,000 fold. Only very small amounts of DNA are required for amplification. RNA can also be studied by first making a DNA copy of the mRNA using reverse transcriptase, this complimentary DNA (cDNA) can then be amplified as above.

Turner PC, McLennan et al. Instant notes in Molecular Biology.
Bios Scientific Publishing. 1997 Oxford University Press.

Question 4

A. false **B.** false **C.** true **D.** false **E.** false

Subcellular organelles:

Nuclei: this contains the bulk of cellular DNA in multiple chromosomes. Transcription of this DNA and processing of the RNA occurs here. Nucleoli are contained within the nuclei: this is where mRNA is synthesized and ribosomes partially assembled.

Mitochondria: Is the site of cellular respiration. Where nutrients are oxidized to CO_2 and H_2O, and adenosine-5-triphosphate (ATP) is generated. They are derived from prokaryotic symbionts and retain some DNA, RNA and protein synthetic machinery, though most of their proteins are encoded in the nucleus. Chloroplasts are structurally similar to mitochondria. See Paper 5 Question 2 for further details of mitochondrial DNA.

Endoplasmic reticulum: the smooth endoplasmic reticulum (SER) is a cytoplasmic membrane system where many of the reactions of lipid biosynthesis and xenobiotic metabolism are carried out. The rough endoplasmic reticulum (RER) is so called because of the presence of many ribosomes. These are engaged in the synthesis of proteins intended for secretion; often these proteins are transplanted to the Golgi apparatus for further modification prior to secretion.

Lysosomes are small membrane – bound organelles which bud off from the Golgi complex and which contain a variety of digestive enzymes capable of degrading proteins, nucleic acids lipids and carbohydrates. They recycle large macromolecules brought into the cell or from damaged organelles.

Turner PC et al. Instant notes in Molecular Biology.
Bios Scientific Publishers. Oxford 1997

Question 5

A. false **B.** false **C.** true **D.** true **E.** false

Calcitriol is produced mainly in the kidney although small amounts are also produced in alveolar macrophages and during pregnancy in the placenta. (See Figure 2).

Calcitriol complements the actions of parathyroid hormone (PTH), its two major sites of action are the intestine and bone. In addition it reduces PTH release by a direct effect on PTH gene transcription.

Figure 2. Production of Calcitriol

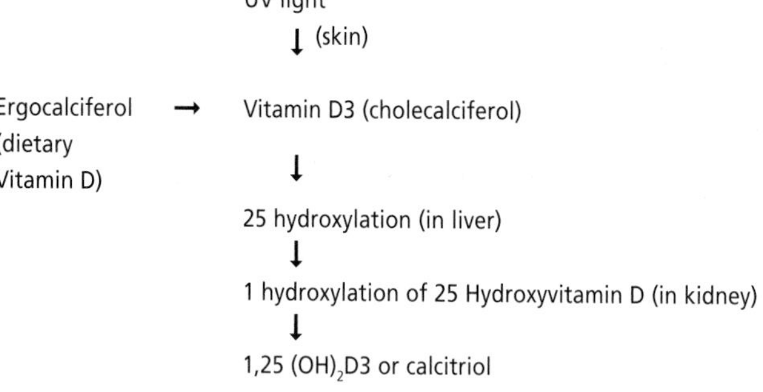

Actions of calcitriol:

1. intestine: increased absorption of calcium
   increased absorption of phosphate

This action occurs by increasing permeability of brush border calcium, promoting synthesis of high affinity calcium binding protein in the cell and accelerating active extrusion of calcium across the basolateral membrane.

2. bone: mainly increases bone resorption

The mechanism of action appears to be increased proliferation and increased differentiation of osteoclast precursors

Calcitriol acts to increase the concentration of ionised calcium and inorganic phosphorous in blood. Production of calcitriol is controlled by PTH, hypocalcaemia and hypophosphataemia (all stimulate 1-alpha-hydroxylase)

Causes of raised 1,25-dihydroxyvitamin D3 (calcitriol):

1. primary hyperparathyroidism
2. pregnancy
3. sarcoidosis
4. rickets (Type II Vitamin D dependent rickets)
5. low phosphate

Causes of a low 1,25-dihydroxyvitamin D3 (calcitriol):

1. malignancy induced hypercalcaemia
2. postmenopausal osteoporosis
3. chronic renal failure
4. rickets (Type I vitamin dependant rickets)

Cunningham J et al. Metabolic Bone diseases
Medicine Souhami/Moxham

Question 6

A. false **B.** true **C.** true **D.** true **E.** true

Water is passively absorbed in the proximal renal tubule. This is in contrast to the following that are actively absorbed through active transport systems:

sodium
potassium
chloride
bicarbonate
urea
uric acid
glucose
amino acids
lactate
phospate
hydrogen ions

After solute enters the glomerulus and filtered in Bowmans capsule it enters the proximal renal tubule. 60–70% of the filtered solute and 60–70% of filtered water has been reabsorbed by the end of the proximal tubule as the filtrate reaches the Loop of Henle. The final 40% of filtered water is reabsorbed in the Loop of Henle (descending limb only), distal tubule (only around 5% as it is relatively impermeable) and collecting tubule. Most of the regulation of water ouput is exerted by vasopressin acting on the collecting ducts.

Ganong WF. Review of Medical Physiology 1999
19th Edition Appleton and Lange Publishers, Connecticut

Question 7

A. true **B.** false **C.** true **D.** false **E.** false

Factors that shift the O_2 dissociation curve to the right (i.e.) facilitating O_2 transfer to the tissues) include:

Raised CO_2 tension / reduced pH (Bohr effect)
Raised temperature
Raised 2,3, Diphosphoglycerate (DPG)

Factors shifting the curve to the left:

Increased O_2 tension
Raised pH / reduced CO_2 tension
Falling temperature locally
Reduced DPG
Carbon monoxide

Increasing the concentration of DPG shifts the dissociation curve to the right, i.e. a state of reduced O_2 affinity. DPG fits into the gap between the two β-chains of haemoglobin when this becomes widened during deoxygenation and also binds to a variety of sites in the central portion of the molecule. As the concentration of DPG rises more haemoglobin molecules are held in the deoxy configuration thus shifting the O_2 dissociation curve to the right.

The metabolic functions of the red cell include:

1. maintenance of Na/K ATPase pumps
2. maintenance of iron in a reduced state by reducing Fe^{3+} to Fe^{2+}, using methaemoglobin reductase (NADH driven)
3. generation of DPG
4. protection of suphydryl groups by maintaining adequate amounts of reduced glutathione
5. synthesis of NAD and NADP

Remember that the O_2 tension in the blood is a function of the amount of O_2 dissolved in the actual blood (outside red cell) not that carried with the Hb molecule. Hence this remains the same in anaemia.

Weatherall DJ Erythropoesis and the normal red cell.
Oxford Textbook of Medicine. Oxford University Press.

Question 8

A. false **B.** true **C.** false **D.** true **E.** false

The primary bile acids cholic and chenodeoxycholic acid are synthesised from cholesterol in the liver, conjugated with taurine or glycine to form bile acids, and excreted into the bile canaliculi and into the duodenum. In the distal ileum they are actively transported across the gut back into the liver. This is the so-called enterohepatic circulation: the whole bile salt pool is recirculated twice in any one meal and the fact that only 5% is newly synthesized in the liver is testament to its high efficiency. 4% of bile salts are lost naturally to the colon but in cases of ileal resection increased bile salts find their way into the large intestine leading to diarrhoea and consequently a reduced colonic absorption of water.

Causes of folate deficiency:

Physiological	pregnancy lactation prematurity growth spurts
Nutritional deficiency	
Malabsorption	coeliac disease tropical sprue gastrectomy extensive Crohn's disease
Drugs	phenytoin
Pathological	chronic haemolysis myeloproliferative disorders severe inflammatory disease dialysis

Folate exists in nature in over 100 forms, all of which are derivatives of folic acid. It occurs in most foods and is absorbed mainly through the duodenum and jejunum. Polyglutamates are deconjugated to the monoglutamates in the intestinal lumen at the brush border.

Malabsorption of B_{12} due to terminal ileal disease occurs most commonly in Crohn's disease, when there is often concomitant iron and folate deficiency.

Other causes of B_{12} malabsorption:

1. Deficiency by intrinsic factor / pernicious anaemia
2. Competition by gut microflora / bacterial overgrowth
3. Drugs e.g. biguanide, high dose K^+ supplements
4. Pancreatic failure possibly by reducing pH and Ca^{2+} concentration of the terminal ileal fluid to below the optimum for absorption

5. Terminal ileal resection

Linch DC. Haematological disorders Medicine
Souhami RL, Moxham J (Eds) Churchill Livingston.

Question 9

A. true **B.** false **C.** true **D.** true **E.** false

The sciatic nerve is the largest in the body and arises from L4, L5, S1, S2 and S3 nerves in the pelvis. It passes through the greater sciatic notch, usually below the piriformis into the buttock. The nerve then runs vertically downward under the cover of the gluteus maximus. At the junction of the middle and lower third of the thigh it divides into the tibial and common peroneal nerves. The sciatic nerve has its own blood supply from the inferior gluteal artery. The nerve supplies all the hamstrings, semitendinosus, semimembranosus and long head of biceps.

Clinical anatomy of nerve lesions in the lower leg:

Nerve	***Site***	***Muscles/ affected limbs***	***Sensory loss***
Femoral	lumbar plexus	quadriceps sartorius	antero-medial thigh and leg towards big toe (saphenous nerve)
Lateral cutaneous nerve to thigh	deep to inguinal ligament	none	outer thigh
Common peroneal	neck of fibula	anterolateral compartment	lateral shin dorsum of foot
Deep peroneal	upper skin	anterolateral	rarely, first web space
Posterior tibial	tarsal tunnel	intrinsic foot muscles	sole

Ger R, Abrahams P. Essentials of Clinical Anatomy
London Pitman Publishing

Question 10

A. false **B.** false **C.** true **D.** false **E.** true

The stem of the question indicates that the problem is a lower motor neurone lesion.

Characteristics of a unilateral upper motor neurone lesion of VIIth cranial nerve:

1. upper face spared
2. tone preserved in lower face

Unilateral lower motor neurone weakness (Bells palsy):

1. upper facial weakness
2. lower facial sagging
3. unable to voluntarily close eyes due to paralysis of orbicularis oculi

Progressively more proximal lesions:

1. between the stylomastoid foramen and chorda tympani leads to the above
2. above the chorda tympani: loss of taste over anterior 2/3rds of the tongue and sensory loss in the external auditory meatus
3. hyperacusis (involvement of nerve to stapedius)
4. above the geniculate ganglion the greater petrosal nerve (motor to lacrimal glands)

Scadding JW, Gibby J. Neurological disease
Oxford Textbook of Medicine. Oxford University Press.

Question 11

A. false **B.** true **C.** true **D.** false **E.** true

Lymphocytes can be divided into two main subtypes: B and T cells both mediate immune reactions. T lymphocytes require the thymus for their development and have a set of surface glycoproteins which are characteristic for them in addition to their own form of receptor. There are two main types:

1. cytotoxic T lymphocytes (these carry the CD8 glycoproteins)
2. helper T cells (that carry the CD4 glycoproteins in mice).

T helper cells (Th) can be divided into Th-1 which release Interleukin 2 (IL-2) and interferon gamma and Th-2 which release IL-4, Il-5, and IL-10.

Helper T cells recognition of an antigen (presented to the T cells by "antigen presenting cells") involves a specific interaction between CD4 and HLA class II molecules. All helper T cells carry this CD4 glycoprotein which measures 55,000Da. Recognition of antigen by T helper cells can be blocked by an anti-CD4 antibody. The CD4 molecule spans the T cell membrane; within the cell on the cytoplasmic side the CD4 is linked to kinase p561ck which has a key role in cell activation. There is evidence that the structure of the CD4 molecule is related to the immunoglobulin superfamily. Low levels of CD4 are also expressed on macrophages and some dendritic cells. CD4 plays an important role in HIV infection where the surface glycoprotein gp120 of the human immunodeficiency virus (HIV) binds to the CD4 therefore acting as a receptor for the virus; HIV shows specificity for CD4+ cells.

The answer to stem a is HLA class II; stem d is B lymphocytes (for expression of IgA).

McMichael AJ. Principles of Immunology
Oxford Textbook of Medicine. Oxford University Press.

Question 12

A. false **B.** true **C.** false **D.** false **E.** true

Histocompatibility antigens are important in man as they play a central role in T lymphocyte function as they can associate with foreign antigen to stimulate T cells e.g. HLA class II +antigen recognised by CD4 cells or HLA class I + antigen such as a viral infected cell recognised by CD8 cells. HLA antigens are encoded by an area of the gene on the short arm of chromosome 6 called the major histocompatibility complex (MHC). There are two types of MHC antigen, class I and II. Most nucleated cells express type I antigen except trophoblasts and only very small amounts are expressed on hepatocytes, muscle cells, and nerve cells. Some tumours are also class I negative which may explain why they escape T cell immunity. Class I molecules on any given cell bind several hundred peptides giving that cell a special identity or signature that can then be recognized by T cells. If foreign peptides are also bound to class I antigens e.g. from viruses infecting cells then T cells can react and destroy the cell. The class I molecule acts to display abnormalities within the cell at its surface. Examples of class I HLA molecules are the HLA-A, HLA-B and (expressed at much lower levels) HLA-C. HLA-E, F and G do not reach the cell surface or appear in only a few cell types.

HLA class II molecules are expressed on B lymphocytes, monocytes, activated T lymphocytes and some epithelial cells and can also by induced in certain cell types by interferon gamma for example in thyroid and gut epithelia. The best-studied series are the DR antigens, (DR BI and DRBx alongside DQ and DP). Class II HLA act to present foreign processed antigen to helper T cells.

HLA and disease associations

Locus	***Antigen***	***Disease***	***Relative risk***
A	A3	idiopathic haemochromatosis	8
B	B5	Behçet's syndrome	6
	B27	ankylosing spondylitis	87
		Reiter's syndrome	37
C	Cw6	psoriasis	13
D	DR2	narcolepsy	>50
		Goodpasture's syndrome	16
		multiple sclerosis	4
	DR3	dermatitis herpitiformis	15
		coeliac disease	11
		Sjogren's (sicca syndrome)	10
		idiopathic Addison's disease	6
		Graves' disease	4
		myasthenia gravis	4
		SLE	6
		idiopathic membranous nephropathy	12
		IDDM	3
DR3 and / or DR4		IDDM	8
DR4		IDDM	6
		rheumatoid arthritis	4
DR5		pernicious anaemia	5

Relative risk is the factor of increased risk of developing the disease by individuals with the HLA antigen.

Mackay I, Rosen FS. The HLA System
N Eng J Med 2000 343;10: 702–709

Marsh SG, Svejgaard A et al. Nomenclature for factors of the HLA system, 2000
Tissue Antigens 2001 Mar; 57(3): 236–283.

Question 13

A. true **B.** true **C.** true **D.** false **E.** false

Hereditary angio-oedema is due to deficiency of the C1 esterase inhibitor. It is an autosomal dominant condition. Once levels of C1 esterase inhibitor drop below a critical level episodic attacks of oedema will occur and last typically for 12–14 hrs. These are not itchy and not associated with urticaria. In addition to the subcutaneous tissues the bowel may be involved leading to abdominal pain and oedema of the larynx can by fatal. Factors that trigger an episode have been documented, for example trauma or dental extraction but often there is no obvious cause. In the absence of C1 esterase inhibitor a high level of C2 kinins is generated leading to increased vascular permeability and oedema. The attack persists until levels of C2 are exhausted following which it spontaneously stops whilst C2 levels slowly build up again. The diagnosis is made by demonstrating a low level of C4 alongside a low level of C1 inhibition. Modified androgens have been shown to help the condition such as danazol or stanozolol (they stimulate the production of C1 esterase inhibitor). Occasionally the side effects of these such as delayed puberty, prevention of pregnancy or abnormal liver enzymes demands a change in treatment with plasmin inhibitor (which prevents the production of C2 kinins) such as ϵ-aminocaproic acid or tranexamic acid. Treatment of severe attacks consists of C1 esterase inhibitor concentrate available in all UK emergency departments or if this is not available by an infusion of fresh frozen plasma.

Factors associated with increased risk of allergic drug reactions:

history of allergic disorders e.g. atopy

hereditary angio-oedema

HLA status	e.g. nephrotoxicity from penicillamine in patients with HLA B8
	or DR3 (HLA DR7 are protected)
	skin reactions with penicillamine HLA DRw6
	thrombocytopenia with penicillamine HLA DR4
	lupus like syndrome with hydralazine HLA DR4

The classical description of urticaria is contact urticaria where there is a weal and flare reaction about 20–40 minutes after contact with a variety of agents such as:

Drugs	e.g. streptomycin, penicillin, genatamicin, aspirin, cod liver oil, horse serum, tetanus toxin, menthol, polyethylene glycol etc
Chemicals	acrylics, alcohols, ammonia, potassium salts, clothing dyes, citric fruits, detergents with and without enzymes, formaldehyde, lindane

Miscellaneous	egg white or yolk, fish and shellfish, various insects giving rise to cotton seed itch, grocers itch, millers itch etc; jellyfish, root vegetables, nuts, spices, pollens, flour etc

Some contact urticaria are IgE mediated (animal dander, saliva, seminal fluid) but most are non-immunological as with the nettle or jellyfish sting. Some ointments used for dermatitis themselves contain a base such as sorbic acid or polyethylene glycol that can cause immediate stinging and slight swelling.

Other causes or types of urticaria: cholinergic, heat, angio-oedema, ordinary urticaria or hives, physical urticaria (e.g. to cold, heat, pressure), familial, papular urticaria. Anaphylaxis results from the rapid degranulation of mast cells and basophils. IgE triggered reactions may result from exposure to antibiotics, insect stings, food allergens, and drugs. This process is an example of a Type I reaction or immediate hypersensitivity, other examples of Type III or immune complex mediated hypersensitivity along with extrinsic allergic alveolitis and glomerulonephritis. Essentially this reaction begins with antibody complexes deposited in a variety of sites e.g. kidney, liver, lungs, skin, vessels, synovia. These complexes are able to bind and activate complement which in turn attract and bind to macrophages and neutrophils causing degranulation with the release of enzymes and mediators. This causes an increase in vascular permeability, swelling and tissue damage. Platelets are activated to release vascular mediators and basophils to release histamine and 5-HT.

Kay AB. Allergy and Allergic disease I
N Eng J Med 2000 344; 1: 30–37

Kay AB. Allergy and Allergic disease II
N Eng J Med 2000 344; 2: 109–103

Question 14

A. true **B.** false **C.** false **D.** true **E.** true

Some clinical syndromes or diseases caused by insects:

1. Anaphylaxis eg bee sting
2. Insect venom allergy (IgE mediated anaphylaxis) eg secondary to hornets
3. Local skin reaction from blood sucking flies eg sand fly

4. Wood dermatitis
5. Airways obstruction eg due to acute layrngeal oedema
6. Pruritis eg in scabies or head lice
7. Arthropod born viral encephalitis
8. Variety of dermatological syndromes eg papular urticaria
9. Dermal myiasis
10. Babesia
11. Mycobacterium ulcerans
12. Sporotrichosis
13. Tularaemia
14. Streptococcus pyogenes skin infection
15. Malaria
16. Human African trypanosomiasis
17. Leishmaniasis
18. Filariasis
19. Schistosomiasis
20. American trypanosomiasis
21. Other viral infections eg flaviviruses such as Dengue and yellow fever

Bell JI and O'Hehir RE. Immune mechanisms of disease
Oxford Textbook of Medicine. Oxford University Press.

Question 15

A. true **B.** false **C.** false **D.** true **E.** true

Normal bowel flora

The stomach and upper small intestine are usually sterile or contain only small numbers of transient organisms such as anaerobes that come from food, saliva or nasopharyngeal secretions. The flora at the other end of the small bowel in the terminal ileum resembles that of the colon. 99% of the faecal mass is anaerobic with Bacteroides accounting for up to 40% (B. fragilis – 4% in faecal flora, 40% in colonic flora; B. vulgatus – 40% in faecal flora, 30% in colonic flora). Bacteroides species are Gram negative anaerobic bacilli (rods) that produces beta-lactamase and are sensitive to antibiotic regimes such as amoxycillin plus clavulinic acid, metronidazole and gentimicin. Despite the very large numbers of anaerobes in colonic contents, during infection the organisms in the bloodstream are usually Gram-negative aerobic rods. However, if the patient has an abscess, Bacteroides or other anaerobes may cause septicaemia. Anaerobic bacteria that cause disease in humans are almost always derived from the hosts own commensal flora (excluding bites and trauma injuries, vertical transmission of anaerobes at parturition etc). Although there are several hundred different anaerobic species known to colonize normal flora in humans only a certain few cause clinical infection and they are not necessarily the most abundant. This may be due to certain virulence factors such as:

adhesins
capsules
lipopolysaccharide
hydrolytic and other enzymes
soluble metabolites and products
growth factors

Surface attachment structures such as fimbriae have been described in B. fragilis and may enable adherence to epithelial cells (important for colonization and infection). Capsules, again described in B. fragilis, confer resistance to phagocytosis, can inhibit migration of macrophages and may potentiate abscess formation. Once septicaemia is estalished for example following perforation other pathologies may ensue such as multi organ failure and Bacteroides as a species cause mortalities in the range of 25–40% in most case series. Other than septicaemia Bacteroides have been implicated in bacterial overgrowth in the small bowel, cholangitis in the clinical setting of gall stones in the biliary tree, rarely in bacterial endocarditis, nosocomial pneumonia, bacterial vaginosis (in conjunction with other species), pelvic inflammatory disease and cerebral abscess.

Many aerobic bacteria are facultative anaerobes ie. they can grow in an anaerobic environment. Clinically this is important in the setting of antibacterial drugs that work by entering bacteria via an oxygen–dependent transport system: aerobic bacteria that are growing anaerobically will be resistant to such drugs. Bacteroides species are true anaerobes.

Patrick, S. The virulence of Bacteroides fragilis.
Reviews in Medical Microbiology 1993. 4, 40–49

Question 16

A. false **B.** true **C.** false **D.** true **E.** false

Clinical features of tetanus:

No wound in up to 15–20% of cases

Tetanus likely to spring from trivial (neglected) wounds

It has been documented to follow burns, ulcers, gangrene, necrotic snake bites, middle ear infections, septic abortions, intramuscular injections with drugs that may casue tissue necrosis (eg quinine) and after surgery

Mild disease: mild muscle stiffness esp in face, all skeletal muscles and muscles of swallowing

Facial expression: eyes partially closed, forehead furrowed, nostrils flared, lips pursed, thinned and stretched and the angles of the mouth downturned, risus sardonicus. This latter expression is rarely like the infamous smile but more denotes pain, anguish and fear

Fever, tachycardia, unstable cardiovascular rhythms, circulatory failure and respiratory or cardiac arrest

Severe autonomic disturbance

Sudden death due to unstable cardiovascular status, hypoxia, excessive vagal activity, sudden rise in core temperature above 41 degrees centigrade, massive PE

Iatrogenic secondary sepsis eg due to line infections with gram negative infections

Prognosis dependent on severity of tetanus:

short incubation and rapid onset – poor prognosis with mortality over 50%

neonatal infection – mortality 60–80%

mortality also rises with increasing age over 70, or delayed admission to critical care

Udwadia FE. Tetanus
Oxford Textbook of Medicine. Oxford University Press.

Question 17

A. true **B.** true **C.** true **D.** false **E.** false

Even in the UK malaria is important, accounting for around 2000 cases per year with an annual mortality of 10. Four species exist of Plasmodium:

P. falciparum
P. vivax
P. malariae
P. ovale

Infection with malaria begins with the sporozoite stage where the parasite is inoculated with saliva from an infected female anopheline mosquito (male mosquitoes do not feed on blood). The sporozoite travels to the liver, enters hepatocytes and multiplies to around several thousand merozoites which are then released to infect red blood cells. The parasite at this stage is visible on stained blood films initially as a ring form and then later as an enlarging trophozoite. After 2–3 days the trophozoites form merozoites (schizogony) which rupture the RBC and infect neighbouring RBCs. P. falciparum differs from the other three in that it expresses proteins on the RBC surface facilitating adhesion to organs throughout the body. The latter parasites therefore are sequestered in areas such as brain, lung, bone marrow, muscle and the gut. The cycle is completed when mature sexual parasites are taken up by female mosquitoes. Sexual reproduction takes place in the mosquito gut. The characteristic fever in malaria is thought to be mediated by cytokine release such as tumour necrosis factor alpha when schizont-infected RBCs rupture. Other symptoms include cough, sweating, anorexia and vomiting with dehydration and jaundice. Generally complications in active infection can be related to levels of parasiteamia of around 4% or greater though they can still take place at undetectable levels. The history may be suggestive of the diagnosis: travel to endemic areas, travel through international airports, needle stick injuries, blood transfusions etc. The blood film is the most important investigation.

Complications of P. falciparum

Encephalopathy
Acute renal failure
Severe anaemia
Adult respiratory syndrome
Pulmonary oedema
Hyperlactacidaemia
Hypoglycaemia
Intravascular haemolysis
Jaundice
Shock

P. falciparum dictates a management that differs from the others: hospital admission is advised for oral therapy with quinine (chloroquine resistance is world wide) and to seek and treat any complications in which case intravenous quinine may be given. The others can usually be treated on an outpatient basis. After quinine a second drug regimen is advised for complete eradication of P. falciparum such as tetracycline, doxycycline, mefloquine or sulfadoxine plus pyramethamine.

Molyneux M. Malaria in Non-endemic areas.
Medicine Tropical Medicine 1997 25(1): 28–31

Question 18

A. true **B.** false **C.** true **D.** true **E.** true

Sickle cell anaemia is inherited as an autosomal recessive trait. It is due to a point mutation in both beta-globin chains leading to the replacement of valine by glutamine on position 9. Sickle cell trait is due to the same abnormality affecting one globin gene. The abnormality in the haemoglobin molecule causes the red cell to sickle during deoxygenation. The sickle cell is more rigid than a normal red cell and accumulates in the microcirculation causing a haemolytic anaemia and tissue infarction. It is common in Africa, the Middle East, some parts of the Mediterranean and India. It gives some protection against plasmodium falciparum. Sickle cell anaemia is associated with anaemia and a reticulocytosis. Target cells and sickle cells are seen on the blood film and there is polychromasia (cells are a different colour).

Complications include:

Aplastic crises especially with parvovirus B19
Splenic sequestration causing profound anaemia and splenic enlargement
Auto splenectomy – usually by adolescence, due to recurrent infarcts
Gallstones
Hand and foot syndrome
Bony crises – precipitated by fever, hypoxia, dehydration and cold
Chronic leg ulcers
Papillary necrosis leading to renal failure
Avascular necrosis
Salmonella osteomyelitis
Priapism
Thrombotic events – lung and cerebral
Polyuria is a well-known complication and can occur in the absence of other renal abnormalities

Sickle cell trait is associated with a normal blood count and a normal blood film. Patients are usually asymptomatic unless put under severe hypoxic stress such as during complications during anaesthesia.

Provan D, Chisholm M, Duncombe A, Singer C, Smith A
Oxford Handbook of Clinical Haematology Oxford University Press 1998

Question 19

A. true **B.** true **C.** true **D.** true **E.** true

Haemolytic anaemia can be divided into inherited or acquired. The acquired group can be further subdivided into autoimmune and non-autoimmune.

INHERITED

Abnormal haemoglobin eg. sickle cell, thalassaemia
Abnormal red cell membrane eg. hereditary spherocytosis, acanthocytosis
Metabolic defect eg G6PD deficiency

ACQUIRED

AUTOIMMUNE
Associated with warm autoantibodies – usually IgG
SLE
CLL
Idiopathic
Lymphoma
Myeloproliferative disorders
Methyldopa
Associated with cold autoantibodies-usually IgM
Lymphoma
Mycoplasma
Infectious mononucleosis
Paroxysmal Cold Haemoglobinuria – IgG
NON-AUTOIMMUNE
Haemolytic disease of the newborn
Transfusion Reaction
Chronic renal failure
Haemolytic uraemic syndrome
Drugs-see earlier list
Mechanical including prosthetic valves and open heart surgery
Accelerated hypertension
Burns
Infections including clostridium welchii and malaria
Wilson's disease
Rheumatoid arthritis

J.L. Burton and C.J. Healey Aids to Postgraduate medicine
Sixth edition Churchill Livingstone 1994

Provan D, Chisholm M, Duncombe A, Singer C, Smith A
Oxford Handbook of Clinical Haematology Oxford University Press 1998

Question 20

A. true **B.** true **C.** false **D.** true **E.** false

Causes of a macrocytosis with normal erythropoiesis are

Hypothyroidism
Hypopituitarism
Liver disease with or without alcohol involvement
Alcohol with or without liver impairment
Pregnancy
Reticulocytosis
Aplastic anaemia
Paroxysmal nocturnal haemoglobinuria
Acquired sideroblastic anaemia (cf congenital which is usually microcytic)

Provan D, Chisholm M, Duncombe A, Singer C, Smith A
Oxford Handbook of Clinical Haematology Oxford University Press 1998

Question 21

A. false **B.** false **C.** false **D.** false **E.** true

Bone marrow failure due to aplastic anaemia is associated with a pancytopenia. Bone marrow aspirate shows an empty marrow ie very few cells. Clinically there is anaemia, bleeding or bruising and increased susceptibility to infection. Lymphadenopathy and hepatosplenomegaly are rare. In response to this the production of erythropoietin is upregulated but the bone marrow is unable to respond.

Causes of aplastic anaemia:

PRIMARY
Congenital eg Fanconi's anaemia
Idiopathic acquired – this accounts for around 50% of cases
SECONDARY
Chemicals
Drugs
Radiation
Insecticides
Some infections
Thymoma
Pregnancy

Provan D, Chisholm M, Duncombe A, Singer C, Smith A
Oxford Handbook of Clinical Haematology Oxford University press 1998

Killick SB, Marsh JC. Aplastic Anaemia: management
Blood reviews 2000 14(3): 157–171

Question 22

A. false **B.** false **C.** false **D.** false **E.** false

Griseofulvin is an antifungal agent. Effective for widespread or intractable dermatophyte infections, it is licensed for use in children and can be given long-term. Pregnancy should be avoided during treatment and for 1 month after the course is completed; males are advised whilst taking the drug to avoid fathering children during and for 6 months after treatment.

Griseofulvin is contraindicated in

lupus
severe liver disease
porphyria

It reduces the anticoagulant effect of warfarin as it is an enzyme inducer.

The best treatment for candidiasis is

fluconazole
amphotericin
flucytosine

Aspergillus infections require treatment with intravenous amphotericin or itraconazole.

Roberts DJ. Onychomycosis: current treatment and future challenges British Journal of Dermatology 1999 141 Supp 56 1–4

Question 23

A. true **B.** true **C.** true **D.** false **E.** false

Selective serotonin re-uptake inhibitors include

fluoxetine
citalopram
paroxetine
sertraline

They have less sedating and fewer antimuscarinic and cardiotoxic side effects than tricyclic antidepressants. Side effects include

headaches
insomnia
anxiety
movement disorders and dyskinesias
tremor

convulsions
hyponatraemia
sexual dysfunction
withdrawal syndrome especially with paroxetine

Spiget O, Martensson B. Fortnightly review: Drug treatment of Depression BMJ 1999 318(7192): 1188–1191

Question 24

A. true **B.** false **C.** true **D.** true **E.** false

Acyclovir is an antiviral agent effective against herpes simplex virus and varicella zoster infections and may also be used prophylactically in immunocompromised patients. It is converted to an active metabolite by herpes simplex virus coded thymidine kinase, inhibiting herpes DNA polymerase and hence preventing viral DNA synthesis. Acyclovir is well absorbed orally and excreted via the kidneys (via glomerular filtration and tubular secretion). It can cause renal impairment if given intravenously. It has to be given 5 times a day orally for 5 days.

The treatment of post herpetic neuralgia is unsatisfactory. Early treatment with acyclovir does not prevent it unfortunately.

Leflore S, Anderson PL, Fletcher CV. A risk benefit evaluation of aciclovir for the treatment and prophylaxis of herpes simplex virus infection. Drug Safety 2000 23(2): 131–142

Shugar, D. Viral and host cell protein kinases: enticing antiviral targets and relevance of nucleosides, and viral thymidine, kinases.
Pharmacology and Therapeutics 1999 82(2–3): 315–335

Question 25

A. true **B.** true **C.** true **D.** true **E.** false

Amiodarone is a class III antiarrhythmic drug though also exhibits class I and II activity. It prolongs the action potential duration and effective refractory period in all cardiac tissues. Whilst it is a noncompetitive alpha and beta-blocker amiodarone has little negative inotropic effects. The half life is greater than 30 days and hence a loading dose is required when given orally or intravenously. It is metabolized by the liver to desthylamiodarone which is also active and accumulates in fat and muscle. Amiodarone is indicated for the treatment of SVT, VT and Wolf Parkinson White syndrome.

The major side effects include

Cardiac – prolongation of the QT interval and hence precipitate torsades de pointes
Pulmonary – alveolitis, pulmonary fibrosis
Hepatic – hepatitis
Neurological – tremor, ataxia, peripheral neuropathy
Thyroid – hypo or hyperthyroidism
Cutaneous – photosensitivity
Eyes – corneal micro deposits
Drug interactions – potentiates effect of warfarin and also increases plasma digoxin levels

Verapamil is a class IV antiarrhythmic agent

Podrid PJ. Amiodarone: Reevaluation of an old drug
Annals of Internal Medicine 1995 122(9): 689–700

Question 26

A. false **B.** false **C.** true **D.** false **E.** false

Sulphonylureas increase the basal and stimulated insulin secretion and decrease peripheral resistance to insulin. Contraindicated in pregnancy, they must be used with caution in liver failure. Weight gain is a well recognized complication as is hypoglycaemia. They have varying durations of action. Tolbutamide is probably the safest in the elderly as it has the shortest duration of action.

Excretion varies between the different agents:

Chlorpropamide is renally excreted
Tolbutamide is excreted via the liver
Glibenclamide and gliclazide involve renal and hepatic excretion

Biguanides decrease absorption from the gut and increase insulin sensitivity. Hypoglycaemia is not a feature but there is an association with lactic acidosis indeed phenformin has been withdrawn on account of this. Lactic acidosis is more likely when there has been an acute reduction in hepatic blood flow, for example after myocardial infarction, pulmonary embolus, or Gram-negative septicaemia, but is also predisposed to by excess alcohol intake or leukaemia. Since the biguanides are largely eliminated (unchanged) by the kidney, renal impairment is a contraindication to their use. They do not promote weight gain. Acarbose is an alpha-glucosidase inhibitor which slows carbohydrate absorption. It is not associated with hypoglycaemia. Unfortunately it is very poorly tolerated due to GI side effects, in particular flatulence.

A fourth type of oral hypoglycaemics is now available. They are PPAR-gamma blockers. The first to be introduced into the UK was troglitazone. This has been withdrawn due to liver impairment. However two newer agents, rosiglitazone and pioglitazone, have recently been licensed for use in combination with other oral hypoglycaemics. They have not yet been licensed for use with insulin or as single agents.

Mudaliar S, Henry RR. New oral therapies for type 2 diabetes mellitus: The glitazones or insulin sensitizers. Annual Review of Medicine 2001 52: 239–57

Question 27

A. false **B.** true **C.** true **D.** true **E.** false

Paracetamol is converted in the liver to, amongst others, a toxic metabolite, N-acetyl-p-benzoquinoneimine. This is inactivated by conjunction with glutathione. In overdose glutathione is saturated and the toxic metabolite binds covalently with sulfhydryl groups within the liver cell membranes causing necrosis. The best guide to the severity of damage is the Protrhombin time (PT).

Clinical features of overdose include:

Nausea and vomiting in the first 24 hours
Most then recover by 48 hours
Liver failure, if it develops, becomes apparent at between 72 and 96 hours.
Acute renal failure can sometimes occur without severe liver failure.

Treatment is with intravenous N-acetylcysteine which donates sulfhydryl groups and hence increases the amount of glutathione available to complex with the toxic metabolite. Patients who are chronic alcoholics and those on enzyme inducing drugs are at greater risk and a lower dose of paracetamol may give rise to liver impairment. The concentration of drug is a poor guide if measured more than 16 hours after the overdose. The overall mortality in untreated patients is around 5%.

Poor prognostic indicators include:

prothrombin time >20 seconds at 24 hours (a peak prothrombin of >180 seconds has a survival rate of <8%)
systemic acidosis at 24 hours
rise in serum creatinine

Current advice is that if fulminant hepatic failure occurs continuous infusion of N-acetylcysteine reduces morbidity and mortality. Some patients go on to liver transplantation.

Management of a serious paracetamol overdose with a delayed INR on presentation:

1. Establish time of overdose singly or staggered, paracetamol level > 4hrs
2. Concurrent risk factors (eg heavy chronic alcohol intake) interpret the UK nomograms with caution if there are co-risk factors and/or the overdose was staggered over a period of time and consider using the 'at risk' line
3. INR (transaminases whether at 400 or 14,000 are unhelpful with regard to prognosis); creatinine, (previous creatinines if impaired), blood gases, urine output (catheterize if necessary)
4. Keep the patient well hydrated, IV fluids (with caution if anuric)
5. IV N-acetyl cysteine (until INR becomes normal)
6. Consider prophylactic antibiotics and antifungals
7. Early discussion with the regional liver transplant unit
8. Consider an anaesthetic escort if transferring a patient to a regional transplant centre with severe hepatic encephalopathy (as the Glasgow Coma Scale approaches 7–8 their airway will become at risk)

Mclain CJ, Price S, Bave S, Devalarja R, Shedlofstkys. Acetaminophen hepatotoxicity. An update. Current Gastroenterology Reports 1999 1(1): 42–9

Question 28

A. false **B.** true **C.** true **D.** true **E.** true

Type I error is when the null hypothesis is incorrectly rejected.

Type II error is when the null hypothesis is accepted when it should have been rejected. A type II error is more likely to occur with small numbers.

The power of a study is the probability that the null hypothesis will be correctly rejected. The power to identify correctly a difference of a certain size can be increased by increasing the sample size. The null hypothesis assumes no difference between the 2 populations. The larger the sample the more likely it is to be normally distributed.

Driscoll P et al. An introduction to everyday statistics -2
J Accid Emerg Med 2000; 17: 274–281

Question 29

A. false **B.** true **C.** true **D.** true **E.** true

Arthropathy is the term used to describe joint disease of any type.

Some common causes are:

osteoarthritis
rheumatoid arthritis
gout
pseudogout
psoriatic arthropathy
connective tissue disorders.

Less common causes of arthropathy are:

amyloidosis
avascular necrosis
Behçets
familial Mediterranean fever
hypermobility syndrome
Forestier's disease
sarcoidosis
relapsing polychondritis

Haemochromatosis is associated with an increase in chondrocalcinosis which is a common cause of arthropathy.

Paget's disease is a disorder of bone remodeling. A raised alkaline phosphatase is characteristic. It is associated with joint pain when the involved bone is close to a joint. It usually affects the spine and pelvis.

Pain in osteoporosis is usually associated with fractures. If fractures are excluded then it may be worth thinking of an alternative cause for the pain such as co-exsistent osteoarthritis.

McHugh NJ. Other Seronegative Spondylo-arthropathies
Medicine 1998 24; 5: 40–43

Question 30

A. false **B.** true **C.** true **D.** false **E.** false

Wegener's granulomatosis is a vasculitis affecting small/medium vessels with granulomatous inflammation. It affects the upper and lower respiratory tracts. Whilst it can also cause glomerulonephritis, in actual fact, any organ can be involved. 45% have lung involvement at the time of diagnosis. The lung lesions are often cavitating. Symptoms include epistaxis, crusting around the nose and deafness. It is one of the causes of a collapsed nasal bridge. It is a well-recognized cause of mononeuritis multiplex. It is associated with a positive cANCA in around 90% of cases. Biopsy of the affected organ shows a necrotizing arteritis and sometimes granulomas. Untreated the median survival is 5 months. Treatment includes cyclophosphamide and steroids and symptomatic/metabolic treatment of associated organ damage eg haemodialysis for renal impairment. Cyclosporin and steroids may induce a lasting remission in about 90% of patients.

Other causes of a collapsed nasal bridge are:

relapsing polychondritis
congenital syphilis

Langforf, C.A: Hoffman G.S Wegener's Granulomatosis
Thorax 1999 54; 7: 629–637

Question 31

A. true **B.** true **C.** true **D.** true **E.** true

Primary antiphospholipid syndrome is characterized by thrombosis and livedo reticularis. It is associated with recurrent miscarriages and recurrent venous thromboembolism and the presence of circulating lupus anticoagulant or antiphospholipid antibodies. These were initially described in Systemic Lupus Erythematosus but they actually occur more frequently when not associated with this disease. The major features of the syndrome are:

Thrombocytopenia
Arterial and venous thrombosis
Abortions
Chorea, migraine and epilepsy
Valvular heart disease
Accelerated atheroma

When associated with livedo reticularis and CVA it is known as Sneddon's syndrome.

Lockshin MD. Future trends for treatment of APS
J.Autoimmun 2000 15; 2: 261–264

Question 32

A. true **B.** true **C.** false **D.** true **E.** true

Hypertrophic obstructive cardiomyopathy is an autosomal dominant disorder with equal sex incidence. Classically there is asymmetrical left ventricular septal hypertrophy causing subvalvular aortic stenosis though the right ventricle can also be involved. There may be associated papillary muscle dysfunction and functional mitral regurgitation. Clinically patients usually present with either angina (with normal coronary arteries), dyspnoea, syncope, or sudden death. Young age at diagnosis and a family history of sudden death are poor prognostic factors. Typical features on clinical examination include jerky pulse, JVP a wave, double apex beat, harsh ejection systolic murmur (only present in 1/3rd), pansystolic murmur, systolic thrill and demonstrable variable obstruction though in the majority of cases physical examination is normal. Beta-blockade is the mainstay of treatment as it reduces the left ventricular outflow tract gradient though it does not reduce the incidence of sudden death. Nitrates should not be used for the treatment of angina in these patients. Atrial fibrillation and ventricular arrythmias are common with the latter occurring in 20% of cases. Amiodarone, flecainide, and dysopyramide are all useful in the long-term management of VT in these patients. Characteristic ECG changes are present in 75% of cases. These include LV hypertrophy with ST and T wave changes, deep Q waves in the lateral and inferior leads, atrial fibrillation and pre-excitation syndromes such as Wolff-Parkinson-White. Diagnosis is usually made by echocardiography which typically reveals ASH (Asymmetrical septal hypertrophy), SAM (Systolic anterior movement of mitral valve), and LV diastolic dysfunction. Surgery is reserved for cases who remain severely symptomatic despite medical therapy as there is a significant mortality from post-operative ventricular arrythmias. Myomectomy is usually performed to reduce the left ventricular outflow tract gradient, often in association with mitral valve replacement.

Julian DG. Disease of the Heart. 2nd Ed. 1998 WB Saunders, Philadelphia.

Question 33

A. true **B.** false **C.** false **D.** true **E.** true

Acute cardiac tamponade is a medical emergency that requires prompt diagnosis and pericardial drainage. Clinical signs include raised JVP with prominent x descent and no y descent. In constrictive pericarditis there are prominent x and y descents. A paradoxical rise on inspiration may occur (Kussmaul's sign). Blood pressure is typically low with peripheral cyanosis and shock. Pulsus paradoxus is due to increased right ventricular filling during inspiration reducing left venticular filling. The heart sounds are soft and there may be a pericardial rub. Oliguria or anuria is common. ECG shows low voltage complexes and occasionally electrical alterans. Echocardiography is diagnostic confirming a pericardial fluid collection with right atrial or right ventricular diastolic collapse due to the pressure of the effusion.

Causes of acute tamponade include myocardial infarction with ventricular rupture, aortic dissection, trauma, uraemia, malignancy, anticoagulation, and acute pericarditis.

Swanton RH. Cardiology 4th Ed. 1998 Blackwell Science Oxford

Question 34

A. true **B.** true **C.** true **D.** true **E.** true

Cardiac myxomas are extremely uncommon and usually diagnosed at echocardiography. They are benign tumours generally attached to the left atrium via a stalk. They are usually sporadic though if occurring in association with endocrine overactivty (esp Cushing's syndrome or acromegaly) and lentiginosis this is called Carney's syndrome. Usual presenting symptoms are increasing dyspnoea, orthopnoea, paroxysmal nocturnal dyspnoea, peripheral oedema, and atrial fibrillation. Systemic emboli occur in 40% of patients. Fever, weight loss, raised ESR and immunoglobulin levels are common due to abnormal protein secretion by the tumour. Clinically left atrial myxomas may cause left atrial obstruction indistinguishable from mitral stenosis. Physical signs are a loud S1, rumbling mitral diastolic murmur, apical systolic murmur, and an audible tumour plop (rare). Pulmonary hypertension occasionally occurs. Treatment is by urgent surgical removal following which recurrence is uncommon except for Carney's syndrome where multiple myxomas occur.

Julian DG. Disease of the Heart. 2nd Ed. 1998 WB Saunders, Philadelphia.

Question 35

A. true **B.** false **C.** true **D.** true **E.** false

A petit mal or absence seizure is the name given to a brief alteration in consciousness associated with classical 3 Hz spike and wave activity on the EEG. It starts in childhood with attacks generally petering out in adolescence. Attacks last a few seconds when the subject stops any activity and stares, usually unaware that anything has occurred. Multiple attacks are usual and parents often simply think their child is daydreaming. Hyperventilation typically provokes absences and can be used diagnostically in the outpatient clinic where asking a child to hyperventilate for 3 minutes will provoke a fit in 90% of affected individuals. There is no structural brain abnormality and children are of normal intelligence. 30% of children with petit mal will have one or more generalized seizures. The treatment of choice for petit mal is Ethosuximide or Sodium Valproate. Carbamazepine is contra-indicated as it can increase the frequency of seizures.

Drug treatment of epilepsy

Seizure type	**Anticonvulsant therapy (1st line)**
Petit mal	Ethosuximide Sodium Valproate Clonazepam
Myoclonic seizures	Sodium Valproate Clonazepam
Tonic Clonic seizures	Sodium Valproate Phenytoin Carbamazepine Lamotrigine
Partial seizures	Carbamazepine Sodium Valproate
Eclampsia	Magnesium sulphate

Panayiotopoulos, CP. Typical absence seizures and their treatment. Archives of disease in childhood. 1999 81(4): 351–355

Question 36

A. false **B.** false **C.** false **D.** true **E.** false

Severe vitamin B_{12} deficiency gives rise to a progressive neuropathy affecting the peripheral sensory nerves and posterior and lateral columns. It is usually symmetrical and predominantly affects the lower limbs causing an alteration in gait and a typical feeling of walking on cotton wool. Initially there is symmetrical (often burning) parasthesia and loss of postural sense causing an ataxic gait. The ankle jerks are absent and later the plantars become extensor. Mental and visual impairment with a central scotoma or optic atrophy may be present. Megaloblastic anaemia may be absent but the serum B_{12} level is always low. The differential diagnosis is usually from other causes of a peripheral neuropathy or multiple sclerosis in younger patients.

Causes of absent ankle jerks and extensor plantars:

diabetes mellitus
taboparesis (tabes dorsalis in conjunction with a spastic paraparesis)
Friedreich's ataxia
motor neurone disease
subacute combined degeneration of the cord (SACD)
conus medullaris
paraneoplastic syndromes.

Causes of B_{12} deficiency:

pernicious anaemia
congenital lack of intrinsic factor
partial or total gastrectomy
small bowel bacterial overgrowth
tropical sprue
ileal resection
Crohn's disease (with terminal ileal disease)
yersiniosis
intrinsic factor receptor deficiency.

Patten J. Neurological Differential diagnosis. 2nd Edition. Springer-Verlag London 1996

Question 37

A. true **B.** true **C.** false **D.** true **E.** false

Chronic subdural haematoma presents with either subacute dementia, focal signs, or signs and symptoms of raised intra cranial pressure (ICP). There is typically a fluctuating course with changing conscious level and neurological signs. Those at high risk include epileptics, alcoholics, the elderly and patients on anticoagulant therapy.

Symptoms and signs of raised intracranial pressure:

headache worse in the morning and on straining or coughing
alteration in conscious level or cognitive function
coma
unilateral or bilateral VI nerve palsies
papilloedema
hypertension
bradycardia.

Patten J. Neurological Differential diagnosis. 2nd Edition. Springer-Verlag London 1996

Question 38

A. false **B.** true **C.** false **D.** true **E.** true

Benign essential tremor is inherited in an autosomal dominant manner most commonly appearing in adolescence and early adult life. Typically there is a fast frequency (6–8/sec) action tremor affecting the upper limbs predominantly though all cases are probably not the same as some display a slower more Parkinsonian tremor but lack rigidity and akinesia. Alcohol and beta-blockers suppress the fast frequency form though slower tremors respond better to Primidone at night.

Causes of tremor include:

Parkinsonism
anxiety
alcohol and drugs
thyrotoxicosis
essential tremor
cerebellar disease
Wilson's disease
mercury poisoning
neurosyphilis.

Jankovic J. Essential tremor: clinical characteristics. Neurology 2000: 54(11 Suppl 4): 521–525

Question 39

A. false **B.** false **C.** true **D.** true **E.** false

Beware the stem of this question: it could equally relate to adults, there are no special features to adolescents. Acute confusional state (delirium) is a syndrome characterized by the abrupt onset of marked attentional abnormalities, clouding of consciousness, disorders of perception, thinking, memory, psychomotor activity, and sleep-wakefulness cycle, and a marked tendency to fluctuations in cognitive performance and behaviour.

The features of dementia and delirium are contrasted below. The most consistent abnormality is a disturbance in attention: patients are unable to sustain attention to external stimuli, are distractable and easily lose the thread of conversations. Severe disorientation in time is invariable. Thinking ability is greatly affected and delusions are common. Illusions and hallucinations are also a frequent feature, particularly in the visual domain. Patients may be restless, excitable, and hypervigilant. Alternatively, they may be excessively sleepy, but usually patients oscillate between these extremes, with a tendency to be more aroused and restless at night. Delirium occurs most frequently in the elderly. Those with the beginnings of dementia are particularly vulnerable. Causes of an acute confusional state:

Any form of metabolic disturbance
Intoxication by drugs and poisons
Drug and alcohol withdrawal states
Infections both intra- and extracranial
Head trauma
Epilepsy (post-ictal states and non-convulsive status)
Raised intracranial pressure
Subarachnoid haemorrhage
Focal brain lesions, particularly if the right hemisphere is involved

The prognosis clearly depends on the aetiology, but if the underlying cause is cured then return to baseline performance can be expected. There are clear differences between delirium and acute schizophrenia, in particular Schneider's first rank symptoms are not found in the former. Illusions and hallucinations do occur, although these tend to be visual in nature.

Comparisons and contrasts between delirium and dementia:

Characteristic	***Delirium***	***Dementia***
Onset	Acute or subacute	Insidious and chronic
Course	Fluctuating with lucid intervals, often worse at night	Stable over the course of the day
Duration	Hours to weeks	Months to years
Consciousness	Clouded	Clear
Attention	Impaired with marked distractability	Relatively normal
Orientation	Almost always impaired for time Place/person often incorrect	Impaired in later stages
Memory	Impaired	Impaired
Thinking	Disorganized, delusional	Impoverished
Perception	Illusions and hallucinations common, usually visual	Absent in early stages, common later
Speech	Incoherent, hesitant, slow or rapid	Aphasic features common
Sleep-wake cycle	Always disrupted	Usually normal

Hodges JR. Dementia; introduction. In Weatherall DJ, Ledingham JGG, Warrell DA, eds. Oxford Textbook of Medicine, Oxford: Oxford University Press, 1996.

Question 40

A. false **B.** true **C.** true **D.** false **E.** false

This has been discussed in Paper 1 Question 41.

Presentations of functional anxiety states:

1. Panic attacks: sweating, palpitations, headaches
2. Presyncopal episodes, visual disturbances, paraesthesia, tetany
3. Fatigue, breathlessness, tremulousness, atypical chest pain
4. Poor concentration, sleep disturbance
5. Feelings of unreality, fear of madness, difficulty swallowing

Diagnosis:

1. High index of suspicion
2. Relief of symptoms with the aid of rebreathing bag
3. Simulated voluntary overbreathing with reproduction of the original symptoms

Psychiatry and Medicine. In Gelder M, Mayou R, Geddes J, eds. Psychiatry, Oxford: Oxford University Press, 1999.

Question 41

A. true **B.** false **C.** false **D.** true **E.** false

Features of mania:

Elevated mood, often inappropriately so; occasionally irritability
Uninhibited behaviour
Increased energy and activity
Expansive, self-important ideas; delusions of grandeur
Impaired insight
Reduced sleep
Increased appetite for food
Increased sexual desire
Increased libido
Rapid speech; rapidly changing topics of conversation (flight of ideas)

Auditory hallucinations are more a feature of schizophrenia-like syndromes than mania, memory impairment should raise suspicions of an organic disorder and suspiciousness suggests a paranoia rather than mania.

Gath DH. Affective disorders. In Weatherall DJ, Ledingham JGG, Warrell DA, eds. Oxford Textbook of Medicine, Oxford: Oxford University Press, 1996.

Question 42

A. true **B.** false **C.** true **D.** false **E.** false

See Paper 1 Question 43 for the negative features of schizophrenia, which include social withdrawal.

Individual symptoms that have been found to be highly specific for schizophrenia and have a high positive predictive value are called Schneider's first rank symptoms. These occur in 70% of patients who meet the full diagnostic criteria for schizophrenia.

Schneiders first rank symptoms:

- Third person auditory hallucinations such as:
  - Often in the form of a running commentary
  - Two or more voices discussing the person
  - Thoughts spoken aloud
- Thought withdrawal, insertion and interruption (alien thoughts being inserted into or withdrawn from persons mind)
- Person's thought being broadcast or read by others
- Delusional perception (a delusion arising suddenly and fully formed in the wake of a normal perception)
- Bodily sensations imposed by some outside agency
- Somatic passivity (Thoughts, emotions or actions experienced as made or influenced by others)

Turner T. ABC of mental health: Schizophrenia. BMJ 1997; 315: 108–111.

Question 43

A. false **B.** true **C.** false **D.** false **E.** false

See Paper 4 Question 2 for a discussion on Marfan's syndrome.

Question 44

A. true **B.** false **C.** false **D.** true **E.** false

In normal subjects the extrathoracic airways, central intrathoracic conducting airways, and the peripheral airways all contribute approximately 1/3rd each to the total airways resistance.

The trachea and major bronchi have thick walls consisting of cartilage and smooth muscle. The subsequent divisions between the cartilaginous bronchi and the alveoli are the bronchioles. They consist of a thin muscle layer with no cartilage.

At the end of normal expiration the elastic recoil pressure of the alveoli is balanced by an intrapleural pressure 0.5kPa below atmospheric pressure resulting in an alveolar pressure of zero.

Respiratory blood flow at rest is approximately 5litres/minute.

West JB. Respiratory Physiology the essentials. 6th Ed. 2000. Lippincott William and Wilkins. Philadelphia.

Question 45

A. false **B.** true **C.** true **D.** true **E.** false

The transfer factor (Tco) is a measurement of the rate at which a gas will diffuse from the alveoli into the blood. It is predominantly dependent on the thickness of the alveolar-capillary membrane and the diffusing capability of the gas. Thus it is useful for detecting parenchymal lung disease. Carbon monoxide is used in clinical measurement.

Causes of a raised Tco include:

asthma
alveolar haemorrhage
left to right shunts
polycythaemia
exercise

Causes of a decreased Tco include:

pulmonary fibrosis
infiltrative disease
pneumonia
multiple pulmonary emboli
pulmonary hypertension
anaemia
emphysema.

Pride NB. Lung Function Testing
Oxford Textbook of Medicine. Oxford University Press.

Question 46

A. true **B.** true **C.** true **D.** false **E.** false

Pathogenesis of cystic fibrosis:

A mutation of transmembrane conductance regulator gene (CFTR) is the principal abnormality; this probably represents a critical chloride channel. The CFTR mutation causes defective chloride transport, which in turn causes increased sodium and water resorption from duct and bronchial lumen. Thick tenacious secretions and sputum result, which leads to high frequencies of Staphylococcus and Pseudomonas spp. superinfection. A point mutation of phenlyalanine at position 508 (delta-F 508), the ATP-binding site, is the underlying defect in 70% of CF patients, the other 30% are due to hundreds of different mutations. The heterozygote frequency of the delta-F 508 mutation (about 1 in 40) has been suggested to reflect evolutionary selection due to increased resistance to V cholerae. Severe phenotypes (such as associated meconium ileus, pancreatic insufficiency) usually imply two defective alleles, eg. Homozygote delta-F 508. The reason for the high salt content in sweat in CF is that chloride is secreted in the gland with a CFTR-independent mechanism, but reabsorption of sodium chloride in the distal end of the duct is impaired.

Features of cystic fibrosis:

Respiratory tract
- Structurally normal lungs at birth
- Recurrent bronchopulmonary infection in childhood
- Finger clubbing
- Haemoptysis; can be massive and fatal
- Breathlessness occurs in later stages
- Pneumothorax
- Nasal polyps
- Bronchiectasis

Genito-urinary
- Delayed puberty
- Male infertility due to failure of development of the vas deferens and epididymis
- Females often develop secondary amenorrhoea

Gastrointestinal
- Steatorrhoea occurs in 85% due to pancreatic dysfunction
- Meconium ileus occurs due to the viscid consistency of meconium
- Rectal prolapse, volvulus and intussusception
- Meconium ileus equivalent syndrome may cause small intestinal obstruction later in life

Liver and biliary tract
Fatty liver
Cirrhosis develops in 5% of patients.
Focal biliary fibrosis
Cholesterol gallstones

Miscellaneous
Diabetes mellitus occurs in about 1 in 10 as a clinical disorder, with about 50% having an abnormal glucose tolerance test
Arthropathy
Amyloidosis
Syndrome of inappropriate secretion of antidiuretic hormone.

Koch C. Hoiby N. Diagnosis and treatment of cystic fibrosis. Respiration 2000 67(3): 239–247

Conway SP. Cystic fibrosis: adult clinical aspects. British Journal of Hospital Medicine 1996 55(5): 248–252

Question 47

A. true **B.** false **C.** true **D.** false **E.** false

Farmers lung is caused by Micropolyspora and Thermoactinomyces species present in mouldy hay, is mediated by a type III hypersensitivity reaction and is associated with precipitating antibodies. It is often considered the prototype of the bronchiolar and alveolar disorders that result from hypersensitivity to inhaled organic dusts. Collectively they are known by the term extrinsic allergic alveolitis (EAA). The underlying inflammatory response is present diffusely throughout the gas exchange tissues and for this reason some prefer the term hypersensitivity pneumonitis. It should be noted that the antibodies presence in the blood are not diagnostic of the condition. Prior to the attacks occurring the patient must first become sensitized to the dust; this may take several weeks to years. Following this the individual may experience repeated episodes of an influenza-like illness accompanied by cough and undue breathlessness some hours after exposure to the relevant dust. Acute attacks are associated with cough, dyspnoea, fever, hypoxaemia and general malaise but not haemoptysis. Crackles, but not wheeze will be present in the lungs. In an acute attack it is more likely that the arterial pCO_2 would be normal or low. A chest X-Ray shows a diffuse alveolar filling pattern.

Some examples of extrinsic allergic alveolitis:

Farmers lung
Caused by forking mouldy hay or other mouldy vegetable material
Antigen: thermophilic actinomyces and Micropolyspora faeni

Bird fanciers lung
Caused by handling pigeons, cleaning lofts or bird cages
Antigen: proteins present in the bloom on the feathers and excreta of birds

Malt workers lung
Caused by turning germinating barley.
Antigen: Aspergillus clavatus

Humidifiers fever:

Caused by contaminated humidifying systems in air conditioners. Usually occurs in factories. Antigen: varieties of bacteria or amoebae (eg. Naegleria gruberi)

Causes of eosinophilia:

1. Parasitic infections
2. Allergic disorders eg allergic rhinitis; other type I hypersensitivity reactions – not EAA (type III)
3. Pulmonary disorders

   Bronchial asthma
   Pulmonary infiltration with eosinophilia:
      Simple pulmonary eosinophilia (Ascaris, Ankylostoma, Trichuris; Drugs – aspirin, penicillin)
      Prolonged pulmonary eosinophilia (similar antigens to SPE, and Strongyloides)
      Asthmatic bronchopulmonary eosinophilia (Aspergillus, Candida)
      Tropical pulmonary eosinophilia (Wucheria bancrofti)
      Hypereosinophilic syndrome
      Polyarteritis nodosa

4. Others such as malignancy (Hodgkins disease, carcinoma, leukaemia), sarcoid, hypoadrenalism, eosinophilic gastroenteritis.

Hendrick DJ. Extrinsic allergic alveolitis. In Weatherall DJ, Ledingham JGG, Warrell DA, eds Oxford Textbook of Medicine. Oxford University Press.

Question 48

A. true **B.** true **C.** true **D.** false **E.** true

Lead poisoning is an uncommon cause of abdominal pain. Atheromatous narrowing of the mesenteric arteries are uncommon, and difficult to diagnose.

Causes of retroperitoneal fibrosis:

Idiopathic
Drug ingestion (Methysergide an anti-migraine drug)
Mediastinal fibrosis
Riedel's thyroiditis
Peyronie's disease
Dupuytren's contracture

It may cause mesenteric insufficiency, and therefore abdominal pain as a result, but generally presents with chronic urinary insufficiency or obstruction.

Abdominal pain in the haematology patient:

Biliary colic from chronic haemolytic disorders
Splenic infarct from sickle cell, CML or myelofibrosis
Vaso-occlusive crisis from sickle cell disease
Acute intermittent porphyria
Paroxysmal nocturnal haemoglobinuria
Hodgkin's disease (may be induced by alcohol)

Features of lead poisoning:

Neurological:	acute: headache, ataxia, fits, encephalopathy chronic: wasting of the small muscles of the hand (peripheral myopathy) weakness (motor neuropathy) pyschiatric sequelae
Joints:	acute: arthralgias chronic: saturnine gout
Renal:	acute tubular dysfunction chronic: gouty nephropathy
Haematology:	acute haemolytic anaemia +/– basophilic stippling chronic basophilic stippling +/– haemolytic anaemia
Gastroenterology:	acute colicky abdominal pain precipitated by alcohol and relieved by palpation or calcium (given IV) chronic: constipation, gingival blue line in adults, premature tooth loss pseudo-obstruction (secondary to neuromyopathy)

Baker LRI. Urinary tract obstruction. In Weatherall DJ, Ledingham JGG, Warrell DA, eds. Oxford Textbook of Medicine, Oxford: Oxford University Press, 1996.

Epstein RJ. Medicine for examinations. 3rd Ed. Churchill Livingstone, London, 1996.

Question 49

A. false **B.** true **C.** false **D.** false **E.** true

Paper 5 Question 50 lists the extra-intestinal manifestations of Crohn's disease. HLA B27 is not more common in Crohn's than the general population. A low-fibre diet may be recommended as a management strategy for those Crohn's patients with stricturing disease. There is a positive association between smoking and Crohn's disease. Conversely 95% patients with ulcerative colitis (UC) are non-smokers or ex-smokers and there is anecdotal evidence that smoking may be protective in patients with ulcerative colitis. Delayed puberty is common in young patients with Crohn's disease. Crohn's disease is associated with Erythema nodosum (EN).

Crohn's disease in focus:

Occurs anywhere from mouth to anus

Symptoms depend on the location of the disease eg ileal disease leading to diarrhoea and weight loss; and colonic disease leading to diarrhoea and rectal bleeding (which is usually painless).

Reactive inflammation outside the bowel: eg acute arthritis, anterior uveitis or EN

Frequency: similar to ulcerative colitis (4 new cases per 100,000 in the UK each year) with a prevalence of 50/100,000.

Predominantly affects whites (black Africans rarely affected at all)

Family history: 10% of patients (35% of which have UC not Crohn's)

Commonest site for disease: ileal caecal region, followed by colon alone

Inflammation: runs deep into the layers of the intestine in contrast to UC. As a consequence strictures, fissures and fistulae are hallmarks of the disease.

Malabsorption is common: leading for example in the very young to diminished growth, nutritional deficiencies and or metabolic bone disease (osteoporosis).

Histology: non caseating granulomata is the hallmark of the disease but is only present in around 30% of histology specimens.

Jewell DP. Crohn's disease. In Weatherall DJ, Ledingham JGG, Warrell DA, eds. Oxford Textbook of Medicine, Oxford: Oxford University Press, 1996.

Question 50

A. true **B.** true **C.** false **D.** false **E.** false

The risk of colonic carcinoma in ulcerative colitis is at its highest by far in those with a history of at least 8 years of pan-ulcerative colitis and in those with primary sclerosing cholangitis. Generally these patients are entered into a local colonoscopy surveillance program. Multiple lesions may be present in the colon, although it is only the adenomas that are pre-malignant. Often the patient is asymptomatic but any symptoms may easily be confused with a flare-up of colitis and so ideally the carcinoma should be diagnosed on a routine colonoscopy as part of a surveillance program.

Gyde SN, Prior P, Allen RN et al. Colorectal cancer in ulcerative colitis: a cohort study of primary referrals from three centers. Gut 1988; 29: 206–217

Byers T, Levin B, Rothenberger D et al. American Cancer Society guidelines for screening and surveillance for early detection of colorectal polyps and cancer: Update 1997. CA Cancer J Clin 1997; 47: 154–160

Question 51

A. false **B.** true **C.** true **D.** false **E.** true

Acute (fulminant) liver failure is characterized by acute liver impairment and altered mentation. Acute liver disease is more likely if the following are a feature:

Short history
Small liver
No spider naevi
Well nourished
Ascites late
Early encephalopathy
Small or absent varices
No identifiable precipitating event

This is in contrast to those with signs of chronic liver disease, a frequent presentation on a typical medical on call take. Acute liver failure is typified by cerebral oedema, severe hypoglycaemia, severe coagulopathy and rapid improvement if the underlying liver disease is reversible. Its usually due to an acute illness such as acute viral hepatitis, poisoning (paracetamol or mushroom), drug reaction (halothane or isoniazid) or fatty liver of pregnancy. The onset of jaundice enables the clinician to classify the type of acute presentation of liver failure as redefined by John O'Grady in 1993

(Kings Liver Unit). The most severe of these (the hyperacute presentation) where jaundice appears within 8 days of the onset of the illness has paradoxically the best prognosis. Management is aimed at the following: identifying a precipitant, preventing hypoglycaemia, avoiding sedation, avoiding aggressive fluid overload which may precipitate cerebral oedema and, whilst nursing the patient in an intensive care setting, contacting the transplant centre early. Guidelines for referral and transplantation take into account the pH, PT (or INR), encephalopathy and evidence of renal impairment.

More than 350 million people world wide are infected with hepatitis B (HBV). This virus is a leading cause of chronic hepatitis, fibrosis, cirrhosis and hepatocellular carcinoma leading to around 1 million deaths annually. Risk factors for infection include sexual activity, injection drug use or occupational exposure, household contact, haemodialysis, transmission from a surgeon, and receipt of donor organs or blood products. The viral genome of HBV is a partially double stranded circular DNA of approximately 3200 base pairs that encode four overlapping open reading frames: S, for the surface, or envelope, gene; C, for the core gene; X, for the X gene; and P, for the polymerase gene. The whole virion, or Dane particle, is a 42nm sphere that contains a core or nucleocapsid that houses the DNA.

Serological changes after infection with hepatitis B virus

HBsAg: surface antigen, appears 3–6 weeks after infection and can disappear after about 3 months if the patient seroconverts. Its presence indicates acute or continuing chronic infection. It may become undetectable in severe (fulminant) infections.

HBcAg: core antigen, is the nucleocapsid that houses the viral DNA. When HBcAg peptides are expressed on the cell surface of infected hepatocytes they induce a cellular immune response that is crucial for killing infected cells. The IgM fraction of the HBcAg is helpful in distinguishing acute from chronic infection.

HBeAg: e antigen, is a circulating peptide that is part of the inner core of the virus. It is modified and exported from the cell and serves as a marker of active viral replication; it is present when there is circulating HBV DNA; it is next to rise after HBsAg, and declines rapidly if the patient seroconverts.

Anti-HBc: core antibody; the first antibody to appear. High titres indicates an acute and continuing infection. May persist for months or longer

Anti-HBe: appears next. Its appearance generally relates to a decreased infectivity, or low risk.

Anti-HBs: appears late and indicates immunity. It is present in those who have seroconverted and in those who have had the HBV vaccination; it can become undetectable in those individuals who have recovered from the infection completely.

HBV DNA: is the best marker of active viral replication and can be detected by PCR.

Delta agent: is an incomplete RNA virus that produces liver disease solely in patients with hepatitis B virus infection, as it requires HBsAg for transfer between liver cells.

Four stages of hepatitis B infection exist: the first is characterized by immune tolerance with surface antigen positivity and large quantities of virus detectable (HBV DNA); stage 2 represents the period of an active hepatitis with diminished HBV DNA levels as the immune response increases against the virus. HBV is not itself cytopathic to hepatocytes: it is the level of an intact immune systems response that determines the extent of cell injury (and thus the possibility of viral clearance). Stage 3 denotes clearance of the virus and only occurs with a successful immune response. Stage 4 is the final stage where HBsAg is undetectable with the emergence of antibody to HBsAg and immunity to the virus. Not all individuals go through all phases and those that do may advance at different times. 95% of infected neonates become chronic carriers (as they have an immature immune system); 30% of children become carriers. Only 3–5% of adults become chronic carriers – the rest have acute infections that will then result in viral clearance.

Disease marker	***Replicative phase***		***Integrative phase***	
	Stage 1	***Stage 2***	***Stage 3***	***Stage 4***
HBsAg	+	+	+	–
Antibody to HBsAg	–	–	–	+
HBV DNA	strongly +ve	+	–	–
Antibody to HBcAg	+	+	+	+
HBeAg	+	+	–	–
Antibody to HBeAg	–	–	–	–
AST/ALT levels	normal	elevated	normal	normal

OGrady JG, Schalm SW, Williams R. Acute Liver Failure; redefining the syndromes
Lancet 1993; 342: 1000

Lee W Hepatitis B Virus Infection
NEJM 1997 337: 24; 1733–1745

Question 52

A. true **B.** true **C.** false **D.** false **E.** false

Acromegaly is due to increased production of growth hormone after puberty. The incidence is around 3 per million. It is seen equally in men and women, may occur at any age and is usually diagnosed in the 4th to 5th decades. It may occur as part of the multiple endocrine neoplasia type 1 syndrome in 6% of cases.

Patients have a slow progression of symptoms and signs, so that diagnosis may be long delayed, but obvious when photographs are reviewed. Symptoms and signs can be characterized into:

1. Pituitary tumour mass

   Headache, visual field defects (bitemporal hemianopia), cranial nerve palsies

2. Hypopituitarism

   Gonadal dysfunction

Other anterior pituitary hormone deficiencies (Prolactin, TSH, ACTH). Posterior pituitary hormones are not generally affected.

3. Excessive GH secretion

   Enlarged hands, feet, head tongue and vocal chords
   Skin: hyperhidrosis, greasiness, skin tags, acne
   Increased interdental spaces, malocclusion
   Carpal tunnel syndrome
   Organomegaly
   Hypertension
   Cardiomyopathy
   Neuropathy
   Impaired glucose tolerance and Diabetes Mellitus.

4. Miscellaneous

   Osteoarthritis, arthralgias
   Neuropathy
   Renal calculi

Thyroid enlargement is due to raised growth hormone levels either directly or as a result of generalised soft tissue mass increase. It may be as a result of low TSH caused by hypopituitarism, but this is uncommon.

Serum IGF-1 concentration is the best screening test for acromegaly. Oral glucose tolerance test will show a failure of serum GH to decrease.

The aim of treatment should be the return of normal GH secretion, abatement of clinical symptoms and signs, reversal of tumour mass effects, and preservation of other anterior pituitary function. In practice cure is defined as a reduction in the serum IGF-I to normal for age and sex and a normal GH response to oral glucose. Treatments include surgery, radiation for persistent disease, bromocriptine, somatostatin analogues eg octreotide.

Thorner MO. Anterior pituitary disorders. In Weatherall DJ, Ledingham JGG, Warrell DA, eds. Oxford Textbook of Medicine, Oxford: Oxford University Press, 1996.

Question 53

A. true **B.** false **C.** false **D.** true **E.** false

The polycystic ovary syndrome (usually known as polycystic ovaries or 'PCO') generally starts at puberty and involves menstrual abnormalities, oligomenorrhoea or amenorrhoea, hyperandrogenization (including hirsutism) and weight increase. Patients do not present with primary amenorrhoea. Many women with PCO are hyperinsulinaemic and there is a strong correlation between menstruation and fasting serum insulin. As a major determinant of insulin secretion is obesity, the deterioration of the menstrual cycle with weight increase and its improvement with weight loss is easily understood.

Polycystic ovaries are generally easily identified by ultrasound scan as they are large (3 times normal), and have cysts of 6–8mm arranged around the circumference. Generally the term polycystic ovary syndrome is used in women who complain of characteristic symptoms in addition to the morphological features.

Women with PCO are not oestrogen deficient; there is extra-ovarian conversion of increased ovarian androgens to oestrogens, mainly in fat tissue, but also in liver and bone marrow. They therefore are not at increased risk from osteoporosis.

The nature of the primary disturbance underlying these findings is uncertain. A central problem is a failure of the ovary to convert androgens, made in excessive amounts by the abundant hyperplastic ovarian stromal cells into oestrogens. Androstenedione (a weak adrenal steroid hormone which mediates the growth of pubic and axillary hair in girls) and testosterone are then released into the circulation and converted in the skin to dihydrotestosterone. In the liver and fat tissue they are converted into oestrogens at a rate which increases with the degree of obesity. The high oestrogen levels inhibit secretion of FSH and may stimulate secretion of LH. The ratio is typically greater than 1:3 respectively.

The hypersecretion of insulin inhibits hepatic synthesis of sex hormone binding globulin (SHBG), which particularly in obese women results in a disparity between circulating testosterone concentrations and the degree of hirsutism. The concentration of unbound testosterone (to SHBG) is very high despite serum total testosterone sometimes being within the normal range, and in these circumstances SHBG levels may therefore be low.

Polycystic ovary disease is not an autoimmune disease. Primary ovarian failure as such may be associated with other organ-specific autoimmune conditions, such as thyroid disease, IDDM, hypoparathyroidism and vitiligo.

Causes of hirsutism:

1. Familial/racial
2. Drug-induced

   phenytoin
   minoxidil, diazoxide
   corticosteroids, cyclosporin A (may strictly be classified as hypertrichosis)
   androgens

3. Adrenal causes, e.g. tumour (causes raised plasma DHEAS/urinary 17-ketosteroids)

   ACTH-inducible rise in 17-hydroxyprogesterone is caused by late onset 21-hydroxylase deficiency (i.e. congenital adrenal hyperplasia)

4. Ovarian origin e.g. Sertoli-Leydig cell tumour (raised testosterone, normal DHEAS)
5. PCO usually LH:FSH >3 plus increased free testosterone (see Paper 2 Question 54)

Jacobs HS. The Ovary. In Weatherall DJ, Ledingham JGG, Warrell DA, eds. Oxford Textbook of Medicine, Oxford: Oxford University Press, 1996.

Question 54

A. false **B.** true **C.** false **D.** true **E.** false

Subacute thyroiditis, probably due to a viral infection of the thyroid gland, often following a respiratory infection, causes follicular destruction from the resulting granuloma formation, with release of preformed hormone, and with biochemical and clinical evidence of hyperthyroidism, i.e. low TSH due to negative feedback and high T4 and T3. New thyroid synthesis is impaired, and once stores of preformed hormone are depleted, clinical and biochemical evidence of hypothyroidism can follow, with a high TSH, but low T4. Ultimately thyroid function usually returns to normal.

Poor compliance with T4 replacement therapy can cause any biochemical or clinical picture, from hypothyroidism, to hyperthyroidism and with low, normal or raised TSH.

Causes of high T4/T3 and raised TSH/or non-suppressed TSH:

1. alterations of thyroid hormone binding proteins
2. drugs
3. intercurrent illness
4. poor compliance with T4 therapy
5. pituitary thyrotrophinoma or adenoma (TSHoma)
6. resistance to thyroid hormone possibly due to:

   structurally abnormal hormone
   reduced accessibility of hormone to tissue due to binding/interaction with another substance
   cell membrane defect
   impaired metabolism of a hormone precursor
   defective receptor for hormone
   post receptor abnormalities

Hormone resistance represents a situation in which inappropriately elevated levels of hormone occur in a setting in which the accompanying biological/clinical manifestations are inappropriate. Most patients with thyroid hormone resistance have generalised resistance to thyroid hormone, and the inheritance is autosomal dominant.

(In TSH resistance the thyroid is resistant to TSH and therefore does not produce T4 in response to raised levels).

A hydatiform mole or choriocarcinoma can stimulate thyroid function, and is thought to be due to high levels of HCG that can be secreted by the tumour. Pituitary gonadotrophinomas would not have this effect.

Early primary hypothyroidism gives either a normal or reduced total and free T4 level accompanied by, and sometimes preceded by, an increase in serum TSH.

Nogueria CR et al. Structural analysis of the thyrotrophin receptor in four patients with congenital hypothyroidism due to thyroid hypoplasia. Thyroid 1999; 9(6): 523–529

Question 55

A. true **B.** false **C.** false **D.** false **E.** true

Ketoacidosis is the hallmark of IDDM. It is caused by previously undiagnosed, and therefore uncontrolled diabetes, interruption or inadequate insulin therapy, or stress of intercurrent illness.

The clinical features relate to: excess fat metabolism to fatty acids with ketone production and osmotic diuresis with large losses of fluid, sodium, potassium and magnesium.

Hypovolaemia, metabolic acidosis and electrolyte imbalance with polyuria then result.

Symptoms and signs are drowsiness, or coma, Kussmaul respiration (deep, frequent hyperventilation), nausea and vomiting. Abdominal pain is a well-recorded symptom of hyperglycaemia, however in the acute admission it should not always be dismissed as part of the syndrome. Hypoglycaemia would cause an increase in appetite. Blood glucose levels may not be enormously high, but are higher than stem 'd'. Plasma bicarbonate is low as would be expected in a high anion gap metabolic acidosis.

Coma need not be present for life to be threatened. Plasma amylase is often more than 3 times the upper limit of normal (usually 1000U/l). This does not indicate pancreatitis.

Singer M, Webb A, Metabolic Disorders, Oxford Handbook of Critical Care, Oxford University Press, Oxford, 1997

Question 56

A. true **B.** true **C.** true **D.** false **E.** true

Severe pruritus is a recognized feature of

- chronic renal failure
- obstructive jaundice
- myeloproliferative disease including polycythaemia rubra vera
- AIDS
- mastocytosis
- carcinoma especially of lung, colon, breast, stomach
- hypo or hyperthyroidism
- drugs
- tabes
- skin diseases including
- dermatitis herpetiformis

scabies
eczema
lichen planus
urticaria

Burton JL, Healey CJ Aids to postgraduate medicine
Churchill Livingstone Sixth edition 1994

Question 57

A. true **B.** false **C.** false **D.** true **E.** false

Rapidly progressive glomerulonephritis applies to cases of acute glomerulonephritis characterized by an abrupt onset and swift decline in renal function over a period of weeks or months. The typical histological lesion is necrotizing crescentic glomerulonephritis usually secondary to antiglomerular basement membrane disease or systemic vasculitis though it can be idiopathic or occur with other systemic diseases. Presentation is generally delayed until the patient becomes symptomatic from acute renal failure with oliguria, peripheral oedema, dyspnoea and uraemia. Urine microscopy reveals an active sediment with dysmorphic red cells and red cell and granular casts. Renal biopsy is essential for diagnosis. On light microscopy the characteristic abnormality is extensive extra capillary crescentic proliferation with a variable number of glomeruli involved. There is proliferation of the endothelial and mesangial cells with narrowing of the capillary lumina and polymorph infiltration of the tuft. The basement membrane may rupture and haemorrhagic necrosis of the capillaries develop.

Causes of rapidly progressive glomerulonephritis

Infectious diseases poststreptococcal glomerulonephritis, infective endocarditis, Hepatitis B, HIV

Multisystem diseases SLE, Henoch-Schönlein purpura, the vasculitides, Goodpasture's syndrome, Essential mixed cryoglobulinaemia, malignancy, rheumatoid arthritis

Drugs penicillamine, hydralazine, allopurinol, rifampicin

Idiopathic or superimposed on another glomerulonephritis (usually membranous or mesangiocapillary type II)

Cotran RS, Kumar V, Collins T. Robbins Pathological Basis of Disease 6th Ed. 1999 W.B. Saunders Philadelphia.

Question 58

A. false **B.** false **C.** true **D.** true **E.** false

Renal involvement is extremely common in SLE with over 50% of adult cases showing clinical evidence of lupus nephritis and nearly 100% showing abnormalities on renal biopsy. In some cases the development of renal disease can predate the development of other manifestations by months to years. Most cases have positive antinuclear factor tests and anti-dsDNA along with a raised ESR and normal CRP. Renal disease usually presents with proteinuria, to nephrotic levels in 50–60%, and occasionally acute renal failure. Frank haematuria is extremely rare. Lupus nephritis can cause virtually any histological lesion from a minimal change to crescentic glomerulonephritis, which the WHO has classified into 5 categories. IgG and C3 are nearly always seen in the immune aggregates and absence makes the diagnosis very unlikely. Treatment should be tailored according to the histopathological type as those with WHO class III and IV lesions require more intensive immunosuppression. Treatment is with corticosteroids alone in milder disease and with the addition of azathioprine or cyclophosphamide in more severe nephritis. There is good evidence that in severe class III and class IV nephritis renal function can be preserved by the addition of a cytotoxic agent in both induction and maintenance therapy.

WHO classification of lupus nephritis

Class	*Microscopy*	*Immunohistology*
I (0–5%)	Normal glomerulus	Scanty mesangial aggregates
II (15–20%)	Mesangial prominence and hypercellularity	Diffuse mesangial aggregates
III (20–30%)	Focal segmental proliferative GN Type (a) limited / (b) diffuse	Diffuse mesangial aggregates
IV (45–60%)	Diffuse proliferative GN with crescent formation	Diffuse mesangial and capillary wall aggregates
V (10–15%)	Diffuse peripheral capillary wall thickening with no proliferation/infiltration	Predominant subepithelial capillary aggregates

Balow JE, Boumpas DT, et al. Management of lupus nephritis. Kidney International 1996 53: S88–S92

Question 59

A. true **B.** false **C.** true **D.** false **E.** false

The combination of proteinuria, hypoalbuminaemia, and peripheral oedema is referred to as the nephrotic syndrome. Urinary protein loss is usually in excess of 3.5g/24h. It is always caused by glomerular disease most commonly secondary to glomerulonephritis, diabetes mellitus, or amyloidosis. Irrespective of cause peripheral oedema can be treated by salt restriction and diuretics along with infusion of salt-poor albumin in severe cases. The complications of the nephrotic syndrome relate to the urinary loss of proteins which is dependent on the selectivity of the protein leak. Infections are common, particularly cellulitis, peritonitis, and pneumococcal infections. Prophylactic penicillin V should be given to nephrotic children and antipneumococcal vaccination considered. Arterial and venous thromboembolism is a common problem with up to 25% of asymptomatic nephrotics showing evidence of DVT on Doppler ultrasonography. Renal vein thrombosis is particularly common in association with membranous glomerulonephritis (6–8% of cases) and investigation is warranted if the patient develops flank or loin pain, haematuria, or an unexpected decline in renal function. Hypercholesterolaemia is present in nearly all nephrotics along with raised LDL and VLDL concentrations. HDL levels are reduced in severe cases.

Causes of the nephrotic syndrome. Glomerulonephritis accounts for 80%, commonly minimal change in children and membranous in adults. Diabetes mellitus, amyloidosis, myeloma, SLE and drugs such as penicillamine account for most of the other cases in the West. In undeveloped countries chronic parasitic infections and malaria are common causes.

Madaio MP, Harrington JT. The diagnosis of glomerular diseases: acute glomerulonephritis and the nephrotic syndrome
Archives of Internal Medicine. 2001 161(1): 25–34

Question 60

A. true **B.** false **C.** false **D.** true **E.** true

Idiopathic retroperitoneal fibrosis is a progressive condition resulting in unilateral or bilateral obstruction at the junction between the middle and lower third of the ureter and is thought to represent an auto-immune peri-aortitis in response to leakage of material from atheromatous plaques in the aorta. This may explain the recognized association of retroperitoneal fibrosis with mediastinal fibrosis and aortic aneurysms.

Retroperitoneal fibrosis is three times commoner in men than women and has a peak incidence between 50 and 60yrs. There is usually a normochromic normocytic anaemia, and raised ESR and CRP. Proteinuria is uncommon. Ultrasound and CT scanning typically reveals the features of urinary-tract obstruction and medial deviation of the ureters.

The differential diagnosis includes lymphoma, carcinoma, and a Crohn's inflammatory mass. Management normally involves a combination of corticosteroid therapy and surgical uterolysis (freeing the incased ureters) or stent insertion.

Drugs causing retroperitoneal fibrosis include methysergide, beta-blockers (esp. practolol), methyl-dopa, and bromocriptine.

Baker LRI. Urinary-tract Obstruction.
Oxford Textbook of Medicine. 3rd Ed. 1996 Oxford University Press. Oxford

Paper 3 Answers

Question 1

A. true **B.** true **C.** true **D.** false **E.** false

When a karyotype is made on patient tissue the chomosomes are laid out sequentially for observation. Types of chromosomal disorders include:

Numerical	***Example***	***Outcome***
Polypoid	69 chromosome	Lethal
Aneuploid	Trisomy 21 Monosomy of X chromosome 47 chromosome	Down's Turner's Klinefelter's
Structural Deletion	Terminal deletion 5p Interstitial deletion	Cri du chat Wilm's tumour
Inversion	Pericentric inversion	Normal phenotype
Duplication	Isochromosome X (fusion of long arm, loss of short arm).	Infertility in females
Ring chromosome	Ring chromosome 18	Mental retardation
Fragile site	Fragile X	Mental retardation
Translocation	Reciprocal	Balanced translocation no abnormalities Unbalanced: spontaneous abortions
Other examples of autosomal abnormalities		Trisomy 18 / Edward's Trisomy 13 / Patau
Other sex chromosomal abnormalities		XXX Triple X XYY XYY male

Pierre Robin syndrome is a disorder of sleep apnoea related to retro or micrognathia in childhood.

Kingston HM. ABC of Clinical Genetics
British Medical Association. BMA publishing

Question 2

A. true **B.** false **C.** false **D.** true **E.** true

Autosomal dominant adult polycystic kidney disease (ADPKD) is the most frequently inherited kidney disorder (1 in 1,000) accounting for 10% of end stage renal failure (ESRF) in the west. It is characterized by multiple cysts arising from various segments of the nephron and involving both kidneys. The mechanisms underlying cyst formation are unknown and to date there is no direct treatment that is curative. Being autosomal dominant the risk of any child is 1 in 2. Penetrance is 100% and new mutations are very rare. The mutant gene responsible for most cases has been located to the short arm of chromosome 16 (PKD1), close to the globin gene. In 15% of families no such linkage is found. A second locus (PKD2) has been isolated in the long arm of chromosome 4. There may very well be an, as yet unidentified, third gene.

Diagnosis rests on: 1) evidence for inheritance and 2) multiple renal cysts in often, enlarged, kidneys on ultrasound. Whilst renal cysts begin in the fetal kidney they are not generally detectable until the age of 20, hence screening does not start before this age.

Presentations vary:

Asymptomatic routine medical, chance finding on abdominal ultrasound but in most cases however patients experience symptoms.
Renal pain due to cyst enlargement, stone or blood clot migration, or bleeding into a cyst
Flank pain bleeding into a cyst
Haematuria
Fever (UTI)
Renal stones occur in 20%; most cases are uric acid stones
Hypertension 30–50% at presentation

Extrarenal manifestations include:

Liver cysts 70%
Mitral valve prolapse 20%
Intracranial aneurysms 4–5% on routine CT screening
Subarachnoid haemorrhage 2–3%
Abdominal herniae are said to be more prevalent

Management includes controlling blood pressure, close follow up of renal function, aspiration of liver cysts under CT guidance, treatment of infection (lipophilic drugs e.g. ciprofloxacin are said to penetrate cysts more easily), dialysis and genetic counselling.

Recessive polycystic kidney disease differs in a number of respects:

1. it is rare (1 in 40,000)
2. neither parents are affected, they are both heterozygotes
3. the mutant gene is on chromosome 6
4. renal cysts occur in the collecting ducts
5. all patients have congenital hepatic fibrosis
6. the disease usually presents in childhood with a variety of presentations:

   hypertension in the first year, gastrointestinal bleeding from portal hypertension, urinary tract infection.

Grunfeld JP. Clinical aspects of inherited renal disorder
Oxford Textbook of Medicine. Oxford University Press.

Question 3

A. true **B.** true **C.** true **D.** true **E.** true

All proteins including haemoglobin undergo a slow, non-enzymatic, covalent formation of aldamine and ketamine sugar adducts at a rate that is related to the local glucose concentration over the lifespan of the protein. In the case of haemoglobin (Hb) the higher and more prolonged hyperglycaemic episodes occur the higher the value of glycated haemoglobin. The shorter the lifespan of the red cell the lower the glycated value will be. Once the red cell undergoes these changes they remain for the lifetime of that red cell. Any protein glycation can be assayed but haemoglobin is more useful than that of fructosamine or albumin for example as the latter have half lives 50% shorter than that of haemoglobin and therefore for oupatient reviews that are spaced more than 2 months apart these protein are less useful.

Lowering the HbA1c level from 9% to 7% over a period of 5–9 years will reduce the incidence of diabetic retinopathy, nephropathy and neuropathy by 50–80%. Conversely low HbA1cs indicate good control with an increased risk of hypoglycaemic episodes. American and European guidelines aim to control the HbA1c below 7% though some bodies maintain that a level below 8% is more easily achievable. Most agree that a level above 8% for 3 months demands intervention. The optimum time interval between measurements is around 4–6 months; and 1–2 months where more strict control is essential for example in pregnancy.

Problems or limitations:

1. Discrepancy of values of HbA1c and blood glucose monitoring

Often due to miscalculation or fabrication of results

2. Low HbA1c due to short red cell survival time eg haemolytic anaemias
3. Expensive
4. Requires in depth patient education

Santiago JV. Monitoring Diabetic Control
Medicine 1997 27–30

Question 4

A. true **B.** true **C.** false **D.** false **E.** true

Chorion villus sampling is a technique where fetally derived chorionic villus material is obtained transcervically with a flexible catheter between 8–12 weeks gestation or by transabdominal puncture and aspiration at any time up to term. Both routes are performed under ultrasound guidance. The risk of miscarriage is around 2% above that of the rate of spontaneous abortions at this time. The main indications include the diagnosis of chromosomal disorders and inborn errors of metabolism.

Amniocentesis is performed at 15–16 weeks gestation. The risk of miscarriage is around 0.5%. About 20ml of amniotic fluid is aspirated directly, with or without local anaesthesia, after location of the placenta by ultrasound. The fluid is normally clear and yellow and contains amniotic cells that are amenable to culture. Discolouration of the fluid may indicate pathology. The main indications for this technique are estimating α-fetoprotein concentration, acetylcholinesterase activity for ? neural tube defects and culturing amniotic cells in those at increased risk of Down's syndrome. The former investigation takes around 7–10 days whereas the latter can take 3–4 weeks. Certain inborn errors of metabolism may also be diagnosed.

Kingston HM. ABC of clinical genetics
British Medical Journal. BMA Publishing

Question 5

A. false **B.** false **C.** true **D.** true **E.** true

The VIth nerve supplies the lateral rectus muscle and arises from the nucleus in the upper pons, ventral to the floor of the fourth ventricle. After passing forwards and downwards it enters the cavernous sinus below the posterior clinoid process. It passes through the sinus and enters the orbit through the superior orbital fissure. A lesion of the VIth nerve causes paralysis of the lateral rectus muscle; this leads to inward deviation of the affected eye and an inability to abduct the eye. The sensory pathway for the corneal reflex is carried in the first (ophthalmic) division of the Vth (trigeminal) cranial nerve. The IVth cranial nerve supplies the superior oblique muscle of the eyeball.

Origins of the cranial nerves

I	Olfactory	forward of the midbrain
II	Optic	forward of the midbrain
III	Oculomotor	midbrain/IIIrd nerve nucleus
IV	Trochlear	sulcus between pons and midbrain at the level of the inferior colliculus
V	Trigeminal	lateral pons
VI	Abducens	medial pons
VII	Facial	sulcus between pons and medulla nucleus in upper pons
VIII	Vestibular	medulla nucleus in lower pons
IX	Glossopharyngeal	medulla
X	Vagus	medulla and cerebellum
XI	Accessory	medulla and cerebellum
XIII	Hypoglossal	medulla and cerebellum

Scadding JW, Gibby J. Neurological disease
Oxford Textbook of Medicine. Oxford University Press.

Question 6

A. true **B.** false **C.** false **D.** true **E.** true

The arm receives its nerve supply from the lower cervical segments C5-C8 and the T1 segment of the thoracic part of the cord. C5,C6,C8 and T1 join together to form the upper and lower trunks respectively and the middle nerve C7 goes it alone as the middle trunk. The trunks then split into anterior and posterior divisions: the three posterior divisions join to form the posterior cord, the upper anterior two divisions form the lateral cord, the lower anterior division continues on its own as the medial cord.

Cords	***Roots***
Lateral cord:	C5 C6 C7
Posterior cord	C5 C6 C7 C8 T1
Medial cord	C8 T1
Nerves	Origins
Axillary nerve	posterior cord
Musculocutaneous	lateral cord
Radial nerve	posterior cord
Median nerve	lateral + median cords
Ulnar nerve	medial cord

The medial cord supplies sensation to the medial side of the arm, forearm and the hand, and through its main branch, the ulnar nerve, the muscles of the medial side of the forearm and the medial side of the hand. Classically the ulnar supplies sensation to the little finger and medial half of the ring finger but not the middle finger. The posterior cord supplies posterior structures, the sensation of the back of the arm, forearm, and proximal hand, and the extensor muscles of these parts. The largest branch is the radial nerve. The radial supplies supinator, and all muscles of the extensor aspect (i.e. extensor and abductors of thumb, extensors of the fingers). It has a minor sensory role only over the back of the thumb and index finger. The lateral cord supplies sensation to the lateral surface of the arm and forearm. The main branch is the musculocutaneous nerve that runs between (and supplies) the anterior muscles of the arm (biceps, brachialis, coraco-brachialis). The median nerve (derived from the lateral and medical cords) supplies the remaining structures, which tend to lie in the midline of the forearm (median) and the part of the hand lying between the medal (ulnar) and posterior (radial) territories.

Ger R, Abrahams P. Essentials of Clinical Anatomy
London Pitman Publishing

Question 7

A. false **B.** false **C.** true **D.** false **E.** true

In 1981 infusion of atrial tissue into rats caused a copious natriuresis hence the term atrial natriuretic peptide (ANP) in stem c. ANPs have a role in protection against hypertension and plasma volume expansion. The natriuretic peptide family currently consists of three peptides:

Atrial peptides

Brain natriuretic peptide

C-type natriuretic peptide

Endothelin, arginine vasopressin, and catecholamines all directly stimulate the release of atrial natriuretic peptide however the dominant stimulus for its release is increased atrial wall tension. Natriuretic peptides exert their effects through binding with high affinity receptors on the surface of target cells. Three types have been described. Receptor types A and B are linked to the cGMP – dependent signalling cascade and mediate many of the cardiovascular and renal effects of the natriuretic peptides. Receptor C is the natural ligand for the B receptor. Type A receptors predominate in blood vessels, B receptors occur mostly in the brain. Both A and B are found in the adrenal glands and the kidney. Binding leads to an elevation of intracellular cGMP.

Actions of Natriuretic peptides:

1. low dose: reduce peripheral resistance and lower blood pressure
2. high dose: increase peripheral resistance despite a decrease in blood pressure
3. increase venous capacitance
4. promote natriuresis to reduce extracellular fluid volume
5. reduce sympathetic tone in the peripheral vasculature through reduction in baroreceptor signals, release of cactecholamines and suppression from the central nervous system.
6. increase renal blood flow
7. reduce renin and aldosterone concentrations

Levin ER. Natriuretic Peptides
NEJM 1998 339: 5; 321–329

Question 8

A. true **B.** false **C.** false **D.** false **E.** true

The baroreceptors can be split into two groups of stretch receptors

1. a series in the carotid sinuses near the bifurcation of the common carotid arteries
2. a series in the aortic arch

Each respond to stretch (or a rise in central arterial pressure) by increasing a salvo of impulses carried by the glossopharyngeal and vagus nerves to the solitary tract nucleus in the medulla and inhibit sympathetic outflow. Efferent fibres are carried in the vagal nerves; the right vagal fibres impinge in the sinoatrial node, the left on the atrioventricular node. In response to a rise in pressure an increase in vagal tone leads to a decrease in heart rate and force of atrial contraction.

The circulating blood volume is kept relatively constant by a combination of factors including:

Atrial natriuretic peptide
Renin – angiotensin aldosterone system
Vasopressin
Osmolality

Renin is stimulated by a local fall in plasma sodium (determined by the macula densa cells) and also by a decreased renal perfusion pressure. Enhanced activity of systemic renin and angiotensin increases aldosterone production leading to sodium reabsorption by the kidney and expansion of the blood volume.

Wilchen DEL. Clinical physiology of the normal heart.
Oxford Textbook of Medicine. Oxford University Press.

Question 9

A. true **B.** true **C.** false **D.** false **E.** true

The four most vasoactive substances produced by the endothelium are:

1. endothelium derived relaxing factor (EDRF) or nitric oxide (NO)
2. prostacyclin (PGL2) both of which are vasodilators, and the vasoconstrictors –
3. endothelin and
4. thromboxane (TXA2)

Vascular endothelium is the main source of PGL2 and in conjunction with other messengers such as nitric oxide and adenosine its very short half life allows for very fine tuning of blood flow for example in coronary flow. An important function is prevention of platelet aggregation and when its production is reduced, for example, by carbon monoxide through smoking, platelet deposition may occur. It has been used as a treatment in primary pulmonary hypertension, severe Raynauds syndrome, acute haemolytic uraemic syndrome and pathological activation of platelets. A reduced synthesis of prostacyclin in conjunction with alteration of the prothrombin complex has been implicated with the so-called lupus anticoagulant in the antiphospholipid syndrome leading to thrombotic episodes.

Hoeper MM. Long term treatment of primary pulmonary hypertension with aerosolized iloprost, a prostocyclin analogue.
NEJM 2000 343: 25; 1866–1870.

Question 10

A. true **B.** false **C.** true **D.** false **E.** true

Causes of hypoglycaemia:

Insulin (exogenous or endogenous)
Drugs – quinine, quinidine, aspirin, beta blockers, pentamidine
Malaria – increased consumption of glucose by malarial parasites, fever, infection, anaerobic glycolysis
Malnutrition
Hypopituitarism
Addison's disease
Cirrhosis of liver and acute hepatic failure
Sarcoma
Severe heart failure or renal failure
Any autoimmune disease
Surgical removal of phaeochromocytoma

Clinical features of hypoglycaemia:

1. adrenergic features: secretion of adrenaline leading to pallor, sweating, tremor and palpitation. Other hormones secreted include glucagon, growth hormone and cortisol.
2. neuroglycopenic symptoms: poor concentration, slow movements, dysarthria, double vision, tingling around the mouth, transient strokes, fits and coma

Aldosterone: a rise in potassium stimulates aldosterone secretion and a fall retards it.

Follicle-stimulating hormone (FSH) secretion: the two principal functions of the gonads in humans are to produce sex steroids and gametes. These activities are controlled by leuteinizing hormone (LH) and FSH which are controlled by hypothalamic gonadotrophin releasing hormone (GnRH) secretion and also in part by circulatory gonadal steroids and peptides as part of a feedback loop. LH regulates sex steroids by Leydig cells of the testis and the ovarian follicles. FSH stimulates gametogenesis and in males stimulates sertoli cells for spermatogenesis.

Calcitonin is produced by the parafollicular (C-cells) of the thyroid in man. Its production is stimulated by a rise in serum calcium and it acts to lower the serum concentration.

Turner RC. Hypoglycaemia
Oxford Textbook of Medicine. Oxford University Press

Wilding J, Williams G. Diabetes Mellitus and disorders of Metabolism
Medicine Souhami / Moxham Churchill Livingston

Question 11

A. false **B.** true **C.** true **D.** false **E.** true

Angiotensinogen is manufactured in the liver. Renin is an enzyme secreted by the juxtaglomerular apparatus and acts on angiotensinogen to release a decapeptide angiotensin I. This is then converted to the active octapeptide angiotensin II in peripheral tissues by angiotensin converting enzyme (ACE) – a high abundance of which is found in the lung.

Aldosterone is one of the major mineralocorticoids manufactured in the adrenal cortex. It promotes uptake of sodium and secretion of potassium secretion in the distal renal tubule. The major control factors of aldosterone production are angiotensin II and extracellular sodium and potassium concentrations.

Angiotensin II is a potent vasoconstrictor which readily increases systemic blood pressure, stimulates the secretion of aldosterone from the zona glomerulosa of the adrenal cortex to enhance sodium reabsorption in the distal tubule, stimulates thirst, and is involved in the glomerulotubular feedback mechanism.

Spironolactone (amiloride and triampterene) all act at the site of potassium secretion on the distal renal tubule promoting a slight rise in sodium excretion but a profound inhibition of potassium secretion. It antagonizes the action of aldosterone, competing for its cytosolic receptor. A consequence of this is the serum levels of renin, angiotensin II and aldosterone increase.

Losartan is a specific angiotensin II receptor antagonist. Unlike ACE inhibitors it does not inhibit the breakdown of bradykinin and therefore the well known side effect of ACE inhibition – a persistent cough – is not a feature.

Whatman AP, Anderson DC. Endocrine disease
Souhami and Moxham (Eds) Medicine Churchill Livingston

Question 12

A. true **B.** false **C.** false **D.** false **E.** true

Cyanocobalamin (vitamin B_{12}) is a complex cobalt containing vitamin that is synthesized by microorganisms; animals obtain it by eating parts of other animals or animal produce (milk, cheese, eggs, etc.), or vegetable foods contaminated by bacteria. Clean vegetables, fruit, nuts, and cereals do not contain B_{12} and cooking has little effect on it. Intrinsic factor, a 49-kDa glycoprotein produced by parietal cells in the stomach, is necessary for the absorption of vitamin B_{12} in the terminal ileum. The intrinsic factor – cyanocobalamin complex becomes bound to receptors in the terminal ileum and absorbed by endocytosis. In the enterocytes, cyanocobalamin is transferred from intrinsic factor to transcobalamin II, another cyanocobalamin-binding protein that transports it in plasma. Deficiency due to lack of dietary sources is rare partly as the bodys requirements are low and also because of its abundance in a variety of foodsuffs. Vegans are at particular risk, however, but even here because of the enterohepatic circulation of vitamin B_{12} they are often able to maintain low levels rather than becoming frankly deficient. If the source of vitamin B_{12} is totally stopped it takes around 3–4 years for deficiency to develop. Problems with absorption are clinically more significant than dietary factors eg defective production of intrinsic factor or damage to the terminal ileum eg in Crohn's disease involving the latter section of the small bowel (60% of Crohn's patients).

Ganong WF. Review of Medical Physiology 1999
19th Edition Appleton and Lange Publishers, Conneticut

Question 13

A. true **B.** false **C.** false **D.** true **E.** true

Like antigen presenting cells, mast cells form another arm to the immune response complementing T and B cell action. Mast cells have a receptor for the Fc portion of the epsilon chain of IgE. When IgE binds to antigen, cross linking the Fc receptors will cause the mast cell to degranulate allowing the release of histamine, kinins, and leukotrienes, which give the typical anaphylactic type of allergic reaction.

Actions of mediators released from mast cells

Bronchoconstriction
Mucosal oedema
Mucus secretion
Chemotaxic and cellular activation

Stems b and c are examples of delayed hypersensitivity (T cell mediated). Mast calls are mostly found in lungs, skin and gastrointestinal mucosa, where one finds the main site of immediate hypersensitivity reactions. T cells play a role in modulating this behaviour. Interleukin 3 (IL-3) is needed for growth, differentiation and survival whilst GM-CSF is antagonistic and inhibits differentiation.

Bell JI, O'Hehir RE. Immune mechanisms of disease
Oxford Textbook of Medicine. Oxford University Press.

Question 14

A. false **B.** true **C.** true **D.** false **E.** false

Type IV reactions (cell mediated or delayed hypersensitivity reactions) denotes T-lymphocytes becoming sensitized by a hapten-protein antigen complex. When the T cells subsequently encounters the antigen an inflammatory response ensues. Examples of Type IV reactions are:

1. drugs e.g. dermatitis caused by local anaesthetic creams, antihistamine creams, and topical antibiotics and antifungal drugs
2. complications as a result of some infections e.g. listeriosis, tuberculosis, leprosy, AIDS (and berylliosis)

Stem a is a type III reaction

Greenwood RM. Hosts response to infection
Oxford Textbook of Medicine. Oxford University Press.

Question 15

A. true **B.** false **C.** true **D.** false **E.** true

Neisseria gonorrhoeae (N. gonorrhoeae) are Gram-negative diplococci of the order of 0.6–1.5 microns in size. Humans are the only host and the bacterium is responsible for a variety of clinical syndromes such as salpingitis, aquired infertility and neonatal blindness. Worldwide the prevalence has fallen (by 95% in homosexuals and 65% in heterosexuals) due to the education in sexual practises following the emergence of HIV and AIDS in the 1980s and 90s. In the UK the incidence of new cases was just over 10,000 in 1994. The current incidence rates around the world is now taken as an indirect measure of the success of HIV education programs.

Spectrum of infection:

Localized:	transitional epithelia eg urethra (male / female) and genital glands (Tysons in males, Bartholins in females) uterine, cervical canal, fallopian tubes anal canal/rectum epididymis conjunctiva pharynx
Disseminated	less than 1% of infections are blood borne majority present as arthritis and dermatitis eg polyarteritis/tenosynovitis involving a variety of joints such as knees, wrists, small joints of the hands, ankles, elbows There is an associated fever and characteristic skin lesion (tiny red papules on distal extremities)
Rare	Endocarditis/Meningitis
Clinical presentations	1. Incubation period around 2–5 days 2. urethral discharge (white, cloudy or purulent) in men symptoms and signs may be negligible and the patient remain infectious for many months 3. Epididymitis/epididymo orchitis 4. Vaginal discharge in females, dypareunia
Diagnosis	Gram stain smear and culture on Thayer-Martin medium PCR
Swabs:	conjunctiva in males and females if indicated, endocervical in women and urethral in males probably give the highest yields for diagnosis Other sites have a much lower yield unless there is evidence of pus or discharge such as anal canal, pharynx, blood, joints, lesions in the skin

When considering treatment culture is important in discerning antibiotic resistance.

Cervical infections are easier to eradicate than either urethral infections in men or pharyngeal infections in both sexes. A variety of agents may be considered for single dose treatment such as third generation cephalosporins eg ceftriaxone or cefixime and fluorinated quinolones such as ofloxacin or ciprofloxacin. Some countries include tetracycline as part of the drug therapy (Chlamydial infection co-exists in up to 45% of individuals). Contact tracing should be undertaken if possible and treatment should be considered for partners.

Phlyctenular conjuntivitis eg as described for tuberculosis in children or ocular sarcoidosis consists of small multiple yellow or grey conjunctival nodules near the limbus in association with a sheaf of dilated vessels.

Judson FN. Gonnorrhoea
Medicine 1996 24; 12: 58–61

Question 16

A. true **B.** false **C.** true **D.** false **E.** false

Some common features of hepatitis A (HAV) and hepatitis E (HEV):

RNA viruses

Route of transmission is faecal-oral

Clinical course consists of clinical (or subclinical) infection with a self limiting hepatitis (patients do not get chronic hepatitis)

HAV is distinguished from the other hepatidides by the fact that viral replication can be achieved in vitro in cultured cells. HAV is associated with areas of poor water sanitation. It is an infection that usually occurs in children: 90% of those infected under 5 years are asymptomatic. Seroprevalence studies in the USA, Japan and Australia suggest that up to 70% of the population have been exposed to it in the past. Although HAV is an enteric infection it is possible to obtain transmission through the parenteral route eg in injecting drug users. Those at high risk include schoolchildren, patients in day-care centres, homosexuals, travellers to endemic areas and sewage workers.

The virus itself is not cytopathic to the cell it infects: the hepatocyte. Liver injury is immune mediated by natural killer cells, virus specific CD8+ cytotoxic T lymphocytes and other cells recruited at the site of inflammation. The incubation period is around 2–6 weeks: the higher the infecting dose the shorter the incubation time. Patients present with symptoms common to any episode of acute hepatitis such as malaise, anorexia, nausia, vomiting and fever. After a few days jaundice becomes apparent and the patient may complain of dark urine and pale stools. After 2–3 weeks the acute illness resolves. Most patients do well however a sizeable minority develop fulminant hepatitis with a mortality reaching 2–3% in some case series. Occasionally the infection is complicated by a prolonged episode of cholestasis which may last up to 4–5 months. Oral steroids have been used in this instance to reduce the hepatitis and shorten this period. Diagnosis is made with a positive HAV IgM. IgM will stay positive for up to 6 months after the onset of the infection. If IgM is negative and IgG positive this indicates past infection; in the presence of positive IgM IgG begins to appear within 1–2 months of the onset of infection reaching a peak at 6 months.

Naoumov NV. Hepatitis A and E.
Medicine 1999 27; 1: 31–33

Question 17

A. true **B.** false **C.** false **D.** true **E.** true

See Paper 2 Question 14.

Question 18

A. false **B.** false **C.** true **D.** false **E.** false

Examples of infection spread by the faecal-oral route:

Enteroviruses
Viral hepatitis (hepatitis A and hepatitis E)
Kaposis sarcoma (in HIV infection)
Bacillary dysentery eg Shigellae
Typhoid
Childhood infections eg Yersinia enterocolitica
Obligate intracellular parasites eg Cryptosporidium Parvum
Giardiasis
Polio

Mayon-White RT. Epidemiology and public health
Oxford Textbook of Medicine. Oxford University Press.

Question 19

A. false **B.** false **C.** true **D.** true **E.** false

On a hyposplenic blood film one would expect to see:

1. Target cells
2. Occasional nucleated red blood cells
3. Howell Jolly bodies
4. Thrombocytosis- this is usually transient but can persist
5. Crenated red cells
6. Pappenheimer bodies (iron granules in siderocytes) – also seen in lead poisoning

Medical causes of a splenectomy include

Coeliac disease
Sickle cell anaemia
Tropical sprue
Ulcerative colitis

Provan D, Chisholm M, Duncombe A, Singer C, Smith A
Oxford Handbook of Clinical Haematology Oxford University press 1998

Frick P. Blood and Bone Marrow Morphology Blood Coagulation, A Manual.
Fourth revised edition Thieme Medical Publishers 1990

Question 20

A. true **B.** false **C.** false **D.** false **E.** false

The direct Coombs test (to investigate haemolysis) detects antibody on the patient's red cells, the indirect Coombs test (for cross-match) detects antibody in the serum.

There are many causes of a direct antiglobulin test:

1. Some drug induced haemolytic anaemias

   Penicillins
   Cephalosporins
   Tetracycline

2. Warm antibody mediated autoimmune haemolytic anaemias

   Secondary to CLL or non-Hodgkin's lymphoma
   Mefenamic acid
   Ibuprofen

Idiopathic
Methyldopa
Procainamide
Interferon alpha

3. Cold antibody mediated autoimmune haemolytic anaemia

Idiopathic
Cold haemagglutinin disease
Infectious mononucleosis
Mycoplasma infections

4. Paroxysmal cold haemoglobinuria

Idiopathic
Secondary to viral infections
Congenital or tertiary syphilis

Provan D, Chisholm M, Duncombe A, Singer C, Smith A
Oxford Handbook of Clinical Haematology Oxford University Press 1998

Question 21

A. true **B.** false **C.** true **D.** false **E.** false

An absolute decrease in the neutrophil count (neutropenia) occurs when the neutrophil count is $< 2.0 \times 10^9$/l. There is an increased risk of infection and the extent of the risk is proportional to the count

1.0–1.5	there is no significant risk
0.5–1.0	some risk
<0.5	major risk: treat all fevers in hospital with broad spectrum intravenous antibiotics

Isolated neutropenia may be the presenting feature in

Myelodysplasia
Aplastic anaemia
Fanconi's anaemia
Acute leukaemia

It can also occur in the following conditions

Post infection – usually viral

Severe sepsis

May be drug induced eg cytotoxics

many antibiotics
NSAIDS
anti thyroid drugs

psychotropic drugs
the count usually recovers within days following cessation of the drug

Autoimmune	haemolytic anaemia SLE in isolation
Felty's syndrome	seropositive rheumatoid arthritis, splenomegaly and neutropenia
Chronic benign neutropenia	
Benign familial neutropenia	
Rare	other hereditary causes eg Chediak Higashi, Kostmann's syndrome

Provan D, Chisholm M, Duncombe A, Singer C, Smith A
Oxford Handbook of Clinical Haematology Oxford University Press 1998

Question 22

A. true **B.** false **C.** false **D.** false **E.** false

Primary thrombocytopenic purpura is due to IgG and IgM antibodies which react with antigenic sites on platelet cell membranes. Bone marrow biopsy shows a compensatory increase on megakaryocytes.

It usually presents with

purpura
epistaxis
menorrhagia
bleeding gums
In less than 1% it presents as an intracranial bleed
Occasionally it is sometimes picked up on a routine blood test.

The condition usually presents in young adults with women more affected than men. It can occur in childhood when it has an acute onset followed by spontaneous recovery in around 90%. In adults <5% resolve spontaneously. Diagnosis is essentially by excluding any other cause as examination is normal. A sub group exists in whom the direct Coombs test is positive – this is known as Evan's syndrome. Most have an underlying condition such as CLL or SLE.

Treatment

1. None if platelet count is >50 and not bleeding
2. Prednisolone at a dose of 1mg/kg/day for at least 3 weeks. Despite a 75% response rate only 15% attain complete remission

3. Intravenous immunoglobulin at a dose of 2g/kg/day over 5 days. Good response but once again only transient
4. Splenectomy for refractory cases (the only proven curative treatment)
5. Immunosuppressive agents are used in those who cannot undergo splenectomy or in the few who do not respond to the surgical procedure

Provan D, Chisholm M, Duncombe A, Singer C, Smith A
Oxford Handbook of Clinical Haematology Oxford University Press 1998

Question 23

A. true **B.** false **C.** true **D.** true **E.** false

Verapamil is a class IV antiarrhythmic agent. It inhibits the slow inward calcium mediated current decreasing AV conduction and therefore blocks intranodal re-entry circuits. It is excreted by the kidneys. Verapamil is contraindicated in heart failure as it is negatively inotropic and in sinoatrial disease. Side effects include:

nausea
dizziness
facial flushing
constipation.

It potentiates the negative effects of digoxin and beta-blockers on the AV node. Verapamil is useful in the management of re-entry SVT and atrial flutter/fibrillation as the increased AV block allows control of the ventricular rate (but it does not chemically cardiovert the arrhythmia to sinus rhythm). Avoid use in the treatment of undiagnosed wide complex tachycardias.

Abernetry DR, Schwartz JB. Drug Therapy: Calcium antagonist Drugs
NEJM 1999 341(19): 1447–1457

Question 24

A. true **B.** true **C.** true **D.** true **E.** false

Alopecia can be caused by heparin. It is non-scarring. The mechanism is unclear.

Angio-oedema is a rare but recognized class effect of ACE inhibitors. They can also precipitate hereditary angio-oedema.

Acne rosacea responds to topical metronidazole or oral tetracyclines. Steroids will aggravate the condition.

Beta-blockers, lithium and antimalarials can all precipitate psoriasis.

Chloroquine is used in the treatment of lupus.

Walenga JM, Bick RL. Heparin induced thrombocytopenia, paradoxical thromboembolism and other side effects of heparin therapy. Med. Clin. North Am 1998 82(3): 635–658

Dillans PI, Coulter DM, Black P. Angio oedema and urticaria with angiotensin converting enzyme inhibitors. Eur. J. Clin. Pharmacol 1996; 51(2): 123–6

Question 25

A. true **B.** false **C.** false **D.** false **E.** true

Drugs known to exacerbate asthma are

beta-blockers
aspirin
NSAIDs

British National Formulary
Published by BMA and Royal Pharmaceutical Society of Great Britain

Question 26

A. false **B.** true **C.** true **D.** true **E.** true

Lithium is used to treat depression, mania, hypomania and bipolar affective disorder. It has a very narrow therapeutic index and requires regular monitoring. Many side effects can occur even in the therapeutic range. These include:

Tremor
Polyuria
Weight gain
Hypothyroidism – this is rare
Nausea
Diarrhoea
Worsening of psoriasis
Interstitial nephritis

Price LH, Heninger GR. Drug Therapy: Lithium in treatment of mood disorders
NEJM 1994 331(9): 591–598

Question 27

A. false **B.** true **C.** true **D.** false **E.** true

This question is essentially asking about enzyme inducers which cause increase metabolism of the oral contraceptive pill leading to breakthrough bleeding or pregnancy.

Some inducers:

Phenytoin
Carbamazepine
Barbiturates
Rifampicin
Alcohol (chronic)
Griseofulvin
Sulphonylureas

Mnemonic: PCBRAGS

Jefferson JW. Drug Interaction Friend or foe?
J. Clin. Psychiatry 1998; 4: 37–57

Vandenbroucke JP. Oral contraceptives and the risk of venous thrombosis
NEJM 2001 344; 20: 1527–1535

Question 28

A. true **B.** false **C.** true **D.** true **E.** false

Metabolic acidosis is a characteristic feature in overdose of:

aspirin
paracetamol
alcohols: benzyl alcohol, ethyl alcohol (ethanol), methyl alcohol (methanol),
ethylene glycol
toluene

Rare causes include:

Inhalation: chlorine, cyanide (and derivatives such as nitroprusside below), formaldehyde, methyl isocyanate

Cardiac drugs: quinidine, calcium channel blockers, sodium nitroprusside

Respiratory drugs: beta-2 agonists, theophyllines, and isoniazid

Meredith TJ et al. Introduction and epidemiology of poisoning
Oxford Textbook of Medicine. Oxford University Press.

Question 29

A. false **B.** false **C.** false **D.** true **E.** false

The standard error is the standard deviation divided by the square root of the number of values. The standard deviation is the square root of the variance.

Variance is calculated by the sum of the values minus the mean divided by the number of observations – 1.

In a positively skewed population the median is greater than the mean thus the standard deviation may be greater than the mean. The student t test is a parametric test as is Pearson's coefficient of linear correlation. Non-parametric tests include Chi-squared, Spearman's rank correlation and Wilcoxon's rank sum test.

Driscoll P et al. Statistics 3: An introduction to statistical inference-3 J Accid Emerg Med 2000 17: 357–363

Question 30

A. true **B.** false **C.** true **D.** true **E.** true

Osteoarthritis is very common. It is the commonest chronic joint disease in the over 65's and is a disease which affects both the bone and the cartilage. There is progressive degeneration of the extracellular matrix which then leads to secondary inflammation. The aetiology is multifactorial. An early feature is fibrillation of the cartilage.

The X-Ray changes seen in osteoarthritis are

osteophyte formation
joint space narrowing
sclerosis and subchondral cyst formation
subluxation in advanced cases

Ellrodt AG et al. An evidence base medicine approach to the diagnosis and management of musculoskeletal complaints. American Journal of Medicine 1997 103(6A): 3S–6S

Lane NE, Thompson JM. Management of osteoarthritis in the primary care setting: an evidence based approach to treatment. American Journal of Medicine 1997 103(6A): 25S–30S

Question 31

A. true **B.** false **C.** false **D.** true **E.** true

Hodgkin's disease is covered in the answer to Paper 4 Question 21.

The adverse prognostic signs in multiple myeloma are severe anaemia and renal failure: if present at diagnosis 50% of patients do not survive 9 months

Chronic granulocytic leukaemia is an illness with a progressive course. Survival is rare at 5 years. It usually presents as anaemia or abdominal pain secondary to splenic enlargement. The white cell count (WCC) is often above 100×10^9/l. Other features include a low NAP score, raised B_{12} and raised uric acid. On bone marrow aspirate the majority of patients are Philadelphia chromosome positive. This is a translocation of the long arm of chromosome 22 to chromosome 9 and is expressed as t(9;22).

Signs of transformation to an acute leukaemia include

symptoms: fever and bone pain
signs: increasing splenomegaly, lymphadenopathy
laboratory: increase in WCC, NAP score
bone marrow aspirate: increased blasts

A lymphoblastic transformation has a better prognosis than a myeloblastic one. 90% of children with ALL respond to treatment and 50–60% are cured.

Poor prognostic indicators include:

presentation at <1yr or >10yr
very high white cell count
males do worse than females
B cell ALL

CLL is a disease which predominantly affects the elderly. In most cases it is an incidental finding on a blood test. 95% are of B cell origin. It does not transform into acute leukaemia. Progression is usually through lymph node involvement, then hepatosplenomegaly and eventually bone marrow failure.

Provan D, Chisholm M, Duncombe A, Singer C, Smith A
Oxford Handbook of Clinical Haematology Oxford University Press 1998

Tirelli U et al. Hodgkin's disease: Clinical presentation and treatment
Cancer Treatment Research 2001 104: 247–265

Question 32

A. true **B.** false **C.** true **D.** false **E.** false

Over the last decade several large multi-centre studies have revealed marked sex-based differences in the treatment and outcome of patients with coronary heart disease. The incidence of heart disease is higher in men than women at virtually all ages and presents clinically at an earlier age. These differences diminish following the menopause but take until the ninth decade to reach unity. Despite this it has now been convincingly shown that the 30-day mortality following myocardial infarction is higher in women. The causes for this remains unclear and controversial though important differences in presentation, co-morbidity, and treatment have been reported. Women generally present later, are more likely to be diagnosed as suffering from unstable angina, are less likely to have ST elevation on ECG, and are less likely to receive thrombolysis than men. In addition they are older and have more co-morbidity in the form of obesity, diabetes, hypertension, and heart failure. Women are then less likely to undergo coronary angiography and angioplasty or coronary artery bypass grafting than men are. Interestingly, women who do undergo angiography are less likely to have significant obstructing lesions than men. Coronary artery bypass grafting also carries a higher operative mortality in women than men. This is probably due to a combination of technical difficulty due to smaller arteries and the presence of co-morbid conditions. Following a successful bypass procedure the long-term outlook for both sexes is the same. Men are twice as likely at any plasma lipid level to suffer from coronary artery disease though the percentage risk reduction from lipid lowering treatment is equivalent for both sexes.

Hochman JS, et al. Clinical presentation and 30-day mortality differ among men and women with coronary heart disease. GUSTO IIb Investigators. NEJM 1999 341: 226–232

Question 33

A. true **B.** false **C.** false **D.** true **E.** false

Causes of myocardial infarction include thrombosis, coronary artery spasm, embolism, hypotension, trauma, aortic dissection, coronary vasculitis (eg PAN, Takayasu's arteritis, Kawasaki disease), aortitis, coronary artery fibrosis following radiotherapy, cocaine, congenital abnormalities.

Viral infection is an important cause of myocarditis which may in turn lead to the development of dilated cardiomyopathy. Other causes include bacterial, fungal, and rickettsial infections, amyloidosis, haemachromatosis, drugs such as alcohol, amphetamines, adriamycin, phenothiazines, carbon tetrachloride, endocrine disorders such as thyroid dysfunction, acromegaly, carcinoid syndrome, diabetes, Cushing's syndrome, phaechromocytoma, Lyme disease, Chaga's disease, and sarcoid.

Julian DG et al (Ed) Diseases of the Heart. 2nd Ed. 1996 W.B Saunders Company Ltd London

Question 34

A. true **B.** false **C.** false **D.** true **E.** false

Supraventicular tachycardia is an imprecise term generally used to mean junctional re-entry tachycardias which are further subdivided into atrioventricular nodal re-entry (AVNRT) or atrioventricular re-entry (AVRT) depending on the basis of the arrhythmia. AVNRT results from the presence of both a fast and a slow atrioventricular nodal pathway. In sinus rhythm conduction occurs via the fast pathway. When this is blocked by a premature atrial extrasystole conduction continues down the slow pathway causing retrograde conduction up the fast pathway setting up a re-entry circuit. The p wave is then buried in the QRS complex as both atrial and ventricular activation occurs simultaneously. Less commonly the antegrade conduction is via the fast pathway and retrograde conduction by the slow pathway resulting in delayed atrial activation shown on the ECG as a late inverted p wave. AVNRT typically presents in childhood or adolescence though can occur at any age. There is no association with structural heart disease and the arrhythmia is generally well tolerated. The usual rate is between 140 and 180b/min and there may be associated polyuria due to release of atrial natriuretic peptide. Vagal manoeuvres including the duck-diving reflex, carotid sinus massage, gag reflex, and valsalva manoeuvre may terminate the arrhythmia and should be taught to patients. Otherwise AV nodal blocking drugs such as verapamil, adenosine, and beta-blockers will terminate the arrhythmia.

AVRT is due to the presence of a distinct accessory pathway with a short refractory period that allows retrograde conduction which establishes a re-entry circuit. A characteristic inverted p wave early in the ST segment allows differentiation from an AVNRT and in sinus rythmn a short PR and delta wave may be present.

Wolff-Parkinson-White syndrome is the classical cause of AVRT where retrograde conduction occurs through an accessory pathway, mainly the bundle of Kent. It has a prevalence of 1–3/1000 in the general population though only 25% develop arrythmias, the most common being an AVRT. WPW consists of two main types dependent on the position of the accessory pathway. Type A denotes a left ventricular pathway characterised by positive delta wave and QRS complex in V1 and negative delta wave in I. In type B WPW the right venticular pathway produces a negative delta wave and QRS in lead V1 and a positive delta wave in I with a negative delta wave in II, III, and AVF mimicking LBBB. AVRT is the most common arrhythmia in younger subjects with WPW though fast atrial fibrillation also occurs and the possibility of an accessory pathway needs to be considered in these cases. Digoxin and Verapamil should both be avoided in WPW as they may accelerate antegrade conduction down the bundle of Kent. Disopyramide, amiodarone, procainamide, and flecainide are all effective in terminating WPW tachycardias by blocking retrograde conduction via the bundle of Kent.

Swanton RH. Cardiology 4th Ed. 1998 Blackwell Science Oxford

Question 35

A. true **B.** true **C.** true **D.** false **E.** false

Innocent murmurs occur in up to 30% of children with the prevalence decreasing with age. These are characteristically ejection systolic murmurs or a mammary souffle or venous hum, have no added sounds, and occur in the absence of structural heart disease. Pansystolic and diastolic murmurs are always pathological.

A third heart sound indicates heart disease in subjects over the age of thirty. It is produced by rapid LV filling. A fourth heart sound is always pathological due to high end-diastolic pressure. T wave inversion in normal adults occurs in 20% in lead V1, 5% in V2 and occasionally in V3 (predominantly in blacks). T wave inversion in V4, V5, and V6 is always pathological. Right bundle branch block (RBBB) may be present in older patients without underlying heart disease but left bundle branch block (LBBB) is always pathological.

Causes of a 3rd heart sound include: mitral regurgitation, ventricular septal defect, post myocardial infarction, ventricular failure, cardiomyopathy, constrictive pericarditis, pregnancy, Paget's disease, thyrotoxicosis, Beri-Beri, anaemia, fever.

Causes of a 4th heart sound include: systemic hypertension, aortic stenosis, HOCM, pulmonary stenosis, acute myocardial infarction.

Ledingham JGG, Warrell DA. Concise Oxford Textbook of Medicine. 2000. Oxford University Press Oxford

Question 36

A. false **B.** false **C.** false **D.** false **E.** false

Motor neurone disease (MND) is a progressive degenerative condition affecting pyramidal neurones of the corticospinal tract (UMN), brainstem motor nerve nuclei, and the anterior horn cells of the spinal cord (LMN) with symptoms and signs dependent on the sites involved. It is commoner in men and with advancing age, being rare before the age of forty. Most cases are sporadic though about 5% of cases are inherited in an autosomal dominant manner, 20% of whom have a mutation in the superoxide dismutase gene. This mutation is only found in 3% of sporadic cases.

The term amyotrophic lateral sclerosis is both synonymous with motor neurone disease and refers to the most common clinical presentation of the disease, occurring in 75% of cases, which involves mixed upper and lower motor neurone signs initially presenting with wasting and weakness of one limb. The co-existence of wasted fasciculating muscles with hyperreflexia and clonus is common and gives the clue to diagnosis. Progressive bulbar palsy refers to patients who present with dysphagia and dysarthria due to a mixture of pseudobulbar and bulbar involvement. Progressive muscular atrophy encompasses the small group of patients who present with predominantly lower motor neurone involvement of the limbs with weakness, muscle wasting, fasciculation, and loss of tendon reflexes. Patients may have overlapping signs and symptoms between the three groups. There is no sensory loss, eye movement disorders or sphincter dysfunction. The disease is irreversible, with a median progression to death of 2.5 years for bulbar onset and 3.5 years for limb onset. The subgroup with progressive muscular atrophy have a slightly better prognosis. In a small number of subjects other clinical features such as extrapyramidal signs, cerebellar signs, dementia, or autonomic system involvement can occur and these cases are commonly termed MND-plus syndromes. Published guidelines dictate that the diagnosis is made on the basis of typical neurological signs, progression over at least 6 months, EMG support of anterior horn cell damage in at least two regions, exclusion of other pathology, and the opinion of two neurologists. The differential diagnosis includes cervical myelopathy, multiple strokes, inclusion body myositis, and X-linked bulbar and spinal muscular atrophy (Kennedy's disease).

Treatment is supportive and needs a multidisciplinary approach. Non-invasive positive pressure ventilation is available for respiratory muscle failure and enteral feeding can be considered for patients with severe bulbar involvement. Riluzole is currently the only drug which has been shown to alter the natural history of the disease by extending survival by 3 months after 18 months treatment though no effect on functional deterioration was seen.

Parton MJ, et al. Motor neuron disease and its management. J R Coll Physicians Lond 1999 33: 212–218

Rowland LP, Shneider NA. Amyotrophic Lateral Sclerosis NEJM 2001 344 22: 1688–1700

Question 37

A. false **B.** true **C.** true **D.** true **E.** true

Memory formation is dependent on the Papez neuronal circuit formed by the medial temporal lobe structures (hippocampus, amygdala, parahippocampal gyrus, rhinal cortex) and the mamillary bodies, thalamus, and cingulate gyri. Any interruption to this circuit can cause antegrade or retrograde memory disturbance e.g. mamillary body damage in Korsakoff's psychosis. Damage to the left neuronal circuit gives rise to a verbal memory deficit where patients are unable to remember conversations, names, or what they have just read, whilst right sided damage gives rise to a visual non-verbal memory loss such as remembering faces. Bilateral damage to the circuit can cause a severe amnesic syndrome where short-term memory is unimpaired but there is an inability to learn new or recall prior events. In general, diffuse pathology such as Alzheimers disease produces global cognitive impairment of personality and memory. Focal pathology usually produces a more restricted deficit without a change in personality or loss of memory until the size of the lesion distorts the anatomy or causes raised intracranial pressure when generalized secondary effects occur. Transient global amnesia is severe amnesia lasting for several hours that normally resolves entirely. Retrograde amnesia occurs at the start of the attack shortening during recovery. The subject is fully conscious throughout and may appear agitated and confused due to awareness of the memory loss.

Causes of severe amnesia include anoxia, hypoglycaemia, herpes simplex encephalitis, Alzheimer's disease, Pick's disease, Korsakoff's psychosis, bilateral temporal lobe infarction, and colloid cysts affecting the III rd ventricle.

Oxbury JM, Oxbury SM. Disturbances of higher cerebral function. Oxford Textbook of Medicine. Oxford University Press.

Question 38

A. true **B.** true **C.** false **D.** true **E.** false

Despite human prion disease being rare, the identification of new variant Creutzfeld-Jakob disease and the increased public awareness mean that the diagnosis is increasingly considered in patients presenting with progressive dementia, psychiatric disturbance or ataxia. There are four known human prion protein diseases. These are Kuru, Gerstmann-Straussler-Scheinker syndrome, Fatal familial insomnia, and Creutzfeld-Jakob disease. Kuru occurred in Papua New Guinea due the passage of infection through ritual cannibalism. Despite cannibalism being outlawed in the 1950s new cases are still arising due to incubation periods of over 40 years though these are now extremely rare. Gerstmann-Straussler-Schneiker syndrome is an autosomal dominant disorder comprising chronic cerebellar ataxia with pyramidal signs and dementia with a more prolonged course than Creutzfeldt-Jakob disease. Fatal familial insomnia is characterized by dysautonomia and progressive untreatable insomnia with late onset dementia.

Creutzfeld-Jakob disease can be subdivided into sporadic, familial, iatrogenic and new-variant.

Sporadic CJD accounts for 90% of all prion disease and usually presents with rapidly progressive dementia, and myoclonus, often with cerebellar ataxia and rigidity. Death usually occurs within 4 months of the onset of symptoms with a mean age of 65. Hereditary CJD is a more heterogenous disease and the clinical presentation varies according to the underlying prion protein gene (PRNP) mutation. Gerstmann-Straussler-Scheinkler and Fatal familial insomnia could now both be considered as different PRNP mutations under the umbrella of hereditary CJD. Iatrogenic CJD resulted from accidental cross contamination during medical procedures that involved tissue with high infectivity such as neurosurgery, corneal transplantation, and the use of human growth hormone. In iatrogenic disease the mean incubation period is 2–10 years for infection by a CNS route and around 10–25 years via a peripheral route such as growth hormone administration. The clinical features resemble sporadic CJD with mean survival from onset of symptoms of 6 months to 2 years.

New variant CJD has a distinct clinical presentation with prominent psychiatric disturbance and depression followed several months later by gradual onset ataxia, cognitive impairment, myoclonus, and dystonia. It was initially identified in 1996 and laboratory transmission studies in mice have shown marked similarity between NV CJD and BSE. It has been proposed that consumption of bovine tissue with high titres of the BSE agent are responsible for the emergence of the disease. To date all cases have had the same PRNP genotype that is thought to confer genetic susceptibility.

Diagnosis of sporadic CJD during life is made on the basis of progressive dementia, typical EEG changes, and at least two of the following features: myoclonus, cerebellar ataxia, pyramidal or extrapyramidal signs, and akinetic mutism.

Iatrogenic CJD is often recognized by the development of symptoms in a patient with a recognized risk factor. New variant CJD should be suspected on the basis of suggestive psychological and neurological features developing in young patients. In the early stages it may be impossible to differentiate from other psychiatric disorders.

Diagnostic investigations

CSF examination reveals a raised protein content but normal cell count. A raised 14–3–3 protein level is sensitive and specific for sporadic CJD but can be raised in other conditions such as encephalitis and stroke. EEG typically shows generalized periodic complexes at 1/sec though in 1/3rd of cases it can be normal. MRI may reveal typical changes in the caudate and putamen in sporadic CJD and in the posterior thalamus in new variant CJD. Brain and tonsillar biopsy can be diagnostic but are often of no benefit to the patient during life.

Will GR. Prion related disorders.
J R Coll Physicians Lond 1999 33: 311

Question 39

A. true **B.** false **C.** true **D.** false **E.** false

Following stroke most recovery occurs within the first 3 months though improvement can continue for 1–2 years. Poor prognostic indicators include impairment of consciousness, urinary incontinence, slow recovery, old age, and severe or haemorrhagic stroke. There is considerable variation in degree of recovery from ischaemic stroke depending on the vascular territory involved which correlates with clinical presentation.

Classification according to the OCSP (see below).

Territory involved	***Mortality at 1 year***	***Dependence at 1 year***
Total anterior cerebral infarct (TACI)	60%	35%
Partial anterior infarct (PACI)	15%	30%
Lacunar infarct (LACI)	10%	25%
Posterior circulation infarct (POCI)	15%	20%

In acute embolic stroke there is a significant risk of haemorrhagic transformation occurring in the infarcted area following anti-coagulation. In these patients gradual oral anti-coagulation is recommended over a few days and heparin should be avoided.

Following stroke there is often transient hypertension due to loss of normal cerebral autoregulation. It generally settles over a few days and anti-hypertensive treatment should not be given unless systolic BP>240mmHg. At this level cautious lowering of the blood pressure over several days can be undertaken but a precipitous drop should be avoided as this can lead to more extensive cerebral infarction

The Oxford Community Stroke Project (OCSP) classified strokes into one of 4 subgroups dependant on the clinical presentation. This correlates with the underlying vascular aetiology, can be used to predict likely outcome, and has good intra-observer reliability.

Refer to original paper for detailed description.

Bamford J et al. Classification and natural history of clinically identifiable subtypes of cerebral infarction. Lancet 1991 337(8756): 1521–1526

Question 40

A. true **B.** true **C.** true **D.** false **E.** true

Medical conditions giving rise to psychiatric symptoms:

1. Neurological conditions

   Cerebral infection eg encephalitis, neurosyphilis, AIDS, abscess
   Cerebral tumour eg primary and secondary eg. Bronchial carcinoma, but psychotic symptoms may be part of a paraneoplastic syndrome
   Others: strokes, epilepsy, Parkinson's, multiple sclerosis,

2. Endocrine and metabolic conditions

   Hypo- and hyperthyroidism
   Cushing's syndrome
   Phaeochromocytoma
   Acromegaly
   Parathyroidism
   Uraemia and dialysis
   Hepatic disorders
   Acute intermittent porphyria (emotional symptoms may dominate; lability and histrionic behaviour are common). Psychosis may resemble schizophrenia. Depression may be a feature with paranoid delusions.
   Vitamin deficiencies eg thiamine; Wernicke and Korsakoff syndromes; niacin and pellagra; B_{12} deficiency (memory failure, confusional states and dementia)
   Drug related psychiatric symptoms; therapeutic and recreational.

3. SLE

Lishman WA. Specific symptoms giving rise to mental disorder. In Weatherall DJ, Ledingham JGG, Warrell DA, eds. Oxford Textbook of Medicine, Oxford: Oxford University Press, 1996.

Question 41

A. false **B.** false **C.** true **D.** true **E.** false

Depression is common in old age, with a prevalence of 10–15%. There are no fundamental differences between the disorder in old age and in younger adults, and the treatment, including ECT is the same. Around 15% do not improve despite treatment.

Symptoms more common in the elderly:

Anxiety and hypochondriasis
Depressive delusions (of poverty, physical illness and persecution)
Hallucinations: obscene, menacing or accusing
Suicide is more likely than in old people

Generally these disorders have a prolonged course, and relapse if not treated for extended periods, often for years.

Although the difference between depressive pseudodementia and dementia itself is an issue, and the two disorders have many symptoms in common, patients with dementia are more likely to suffer from affective disorders than the general population.

Rothschild AJ. The diagnosis and treatment of late-life depression Journal of Clinical Psychiatry. 57 Suppl 5: 5–11, 1996

Whooley MA, Simon GE. Managing depression in medical outpatients NEJM 2000 343: 26; 1942–1950

Question 42

A. true **B.** true **C.** false **D.** false **E.** true

Associations with increased risk of adolescent psychiatric disorder

Heredity

Physical disease, especially in brain damage

Environment ie family factors such as:

Prolonged absence or loss of parent
Separation
Parental illness, particularly psychiatric disorder
Parental discord and open discord between family members
Personality disorder of parent
Large family size
Child abuse and neglect
High level of expressed emotion
Social and cultural factors such as: school influence, peer group behaviour, poor amenities and overcrowding, lack of community involvement

Child and adolescent psychiatry. In Gelder M, Mayou R, Geddes J, eds. Psychiatry, Oxford: Oxford University Press, 1999.

Question 43

A. true **B.** false **C.** false **D.** true **E.** true

Questions about anxiety attacks are common. Anxiety attacks and hyperventilation are commonly encountered in everyday practise and it is important to be able to distinguish them from organic disease.

Physical symptoms of anxiety disorder:

Gastrointestinal eg dry mouth, dysphagia, abdominal pain
Respiratory eg tightness of chest, inability to take a deep breath, overbreathing
Cardiovascular eg chest pain, palpitations
Neuromuscular eg tremor, paraesthesiae, tinnitus, dizziness, headache
Genitourinary eg frequent or urgent micturition; generally nocturia is a sign of organic disease, amenorrhoea

Rotational vertigo is also more suggestive of organic disorder, although generalized non-specific dizziness is common.

Anxiety and Obsessional disorders. In: Gelder MG, Gath D, Mayou R. Oxford Textbook of Psychiatry (3rd edition). Oxford University Press.

Question 44

A. true **B.** false **C.** false **D.** true **E.** false

Flu-like and systemic symptoms are often part of the early symptomatology of Mycoplasma pneumoniae, although the organism does not usually cause pleurisy. Mycoplasma is one of the atypical pneumonias, so called originally because they did not respond to penicillin and were milder than usual. Also characteristically the chest radiograph will have more florid signs than would be expected from the physical examination.

The organism is not diagnosed by gram stain, but is usually detected by serology or detection of cold agglutinins although DNA polymerase chain reaction may prove to be useful.

Manifestations of Mycoplasma pneumonia infection:

Pulmonary
- Pneumonia
- Acute bronchitis
- Bronchiolitis
- Bronchiectasis

Haematological
- Haemolytic anaemia
- Thrombotic thrombocytopenic purpura

Ophthalmic
- Conjunctivitis
- Optic disc swelling
- Optic nerve atrophy
- Retinal exudates and haemorrhages
- Cranial nerve palsies have been infrequently reported
- Optic papillitis

Miscellaneous:
- Pericarditis
- Transverse myelitis
- Bullous myringitis
- Guillain-Barré syndrome

Cold autoimmune haemolytic anaemias are caused by cold agglutinins or IgM antibodies to complement components, give a weakly positive Coombs test, and are associated with Mycoplasma, lymphomas and paroxysmal cold haemoglobinuria.

Warm autoimmune haemolytic anaemias are caused by IgG antibodies to Rhesus components and give a strongly positive Coombs test and are associated with autoimmune disease such as SLE, lymphomas, CLL, Hodgkins, carcinomas and also with drugs, eg. methyldopa.

Chan ED. et al. Mycoplasma pneumoniae-associated bronchiolitis causing severe restrictive lung disease in adults: report of three cases and literature review.
Chest 1999 115(4): 1188–1194,

Question 45

A. true **B.** true **C.** false **D.** true **E.** false

The prevalence of sleep apnoea-hypopnoea or obstructive sleep apnoea is correct, and obesity is not the only association.

Aetiology of sleep apnoea-hypopnoea syndrome:

Obesity
Sedatives; benzodiazepines, opiates
Alcohol ingestion
Intra pharyngeal anatomical abnormalities
Micrognathia
Nasal obstruction
Hypothyroidism
Acromegaly

Presenting features of sleep apnoea-hypopnoea syndrome:

Snoring
Insomnia
Nocturnal choking and/or panic attacks
Hypnagogic hallucinations
Nightmares
Unrefreshing sleep

Other symptoms:

Disorientation after waking
Daytime somnolence
Morning headaches
Depression and personality change
Impotence
Nocturnal enuresis
Decreased libido

Some features may be related to the aetiology, such as myxoedema.

Complications of sleep apnoea-hypopnoea syndrome:

- Psychiatric
  - Depression
- Left ventricular
  - Left ventricular hypertrophy
  - Dilated cardiomyopathy
- Ischaemic heart disease
  - Myocardial infarction
  - Nocturnal arrhythmias
  - Unexpected death during sleep
- Other cardiovascular sequelae:
  - Systemic and Pulmonary Hypertension
  - Cor pulmonale
  - Polycythaemia

Arterial desaturation whilst asleep seems to be responsible for many of the clinical manifestations; generally hypercapnia awake does not seem to occur. The hypersomnolence related to sleep apnoea-hypopnoea causes an increase in the accident rate amongst car-drivers. Lorry-drivers often fall into more than one of the at-risk groups, and are a particular cause for concern. Although there has in the past been considerable enthusiasm for surgical treatment, this is currently waning except in the small proportion of patients who have identifiable anatomical causes. Nasal continuous positive airways pressure (CPAP) is currently the gold standard.

JR Stradling. Sleep-related disorders of breathing. In Weatherall DJ, Ledingham JGG, Warrell DA, eds. Oxford Textbook of Medicine. Oxford University Press.

Question 46

A. false **B.** true **C.** false **D.** false **E.** false

CT scan can assess operability in lung cancer by determining if there is mediastinal spread and the extent, if any, of lymph node spread.

Pneumonectomy is not undertaken in patients who cannot sustain an FEV1 of more than 1.2 litres. In a patient with no clinical or biochemical features to suggest metastases (T3, N2 or M1 disease) a thoracotomy would be undertaken, providing that chest radiography, any pleural effusion cytology, CT scan and, if necessary mediastinoscopy were not contraindicative.

Sputum cytology, differential perfusion scan and total lung capacity are not used to assess the appropriateness of surgery in patients where there are no other signs of spread. Isotope scans, abdominal CT and more sophisticated tests would only be carried out if there were a suspicion from clinical or biochemical evidence.

Deslauriers J. Gregoire J. Surgical therapy of early non-small cell lung cancer. Chest. 2000 117(4) Supp 1: 104S–109S

Epstein RJ. Medicine for examinations. 3rd Ed. Churchill Livingstone, London, 1996.

Question 47

A. true **B.** false **C.** false **D.** true **E.** true

It is likely that the above patient has Syndrome of Inappropriate Antidiuretic Hormone Secretion (SIADH) due to his, probably small cell, bronchial carcinoma. His fits may be due to his hyponatraemia, although careful consideration to other causes should be considered, as a serum sodium at this level, particularly if arrived at slowly, would not always cause such severe symptoms. Generally the development of symptoms is more dependent on the rate of decline of the sodium rather than the absolute level.

Weight gain, hypertension and oedema are not generally features, despite the hypervolaemia, although elderly patients may develop heart failure. Measurement of plasma vasopressin is not helpful.

The important differential diagnoses to exclude are myxoedema, Addison's disease (look for the raised K+) and chlorpropamide use.

Diagnosis of SIADH rests on a plasma osmolality of less than 275mosm/L, an inappropriately high urinary osmolality and a urinary sodium greater than 20.

Treatment options include:

Treatment of underlying cause
Water restriction and/or frusemide
Demeclocycline
Hypertonic saline (NB – may precipitate heart failure or cerebral oedema)

Causes of SIADH:

CNS Disorders
Skull fracture
Subdural or subarachnoid haemorrhage
Stroke
Cerebral atrophy
Acute encephalitis
Bacterial or Tuberculous meningitis

Porphyria
Guillain-Barré syndrome

Non-malignant pulmonary diseases
Tuberculosis
Lung abscess/ Empyema
Pneumonia
Chronic obstructive pulmonary disease
Cystic fibrosis (probably related to the above)

Malignant neoplasms with autonomous ADH secretion
Small cell carcinoma of the lung (most common association)
Pancreatic carcinoma
Duodenal carcinoma
Thymoma

Drugs
Chlorpropamide
Vinca-alkaloids
Cyclophosphamide
Carbamazepine
Oxytocin
Narcotics
Tricyclic anti-depressants

Miscellaneous
Hypothyroidism
Positive pressure ventilation

Wilson JD. Endocrinology and Metabolism. In Isselbacher KJ, Braunwald E, Wilson JD et al., eds. Harrisons Principles of Internal Medicine, 13th Edition. New York: McGraw-Hill, 1994
Adrogue HJ, Madias NE. Hyponatraemia
NEJM 2000 342: 21: 1581–1589

Question 48

A. true **B.** false **C.** false **D.** true **E.** false

The normal portal venous pressure is about 10mmHg, but rises to 20–40mmHG in portal hypertension. The causes of portal hypertension can be classified as

1. Presinusoidal (ie on the portal side of the liver) where the hepatic vein wedge pressure is low or normal as there is no resistance to the flow of blood towards the liver
2. Sinusoidal where the wedge pressure is raised and reflects the portal pressure.

3. Post sinusoidal (on the hepatic venous side of the liver). Here the pressure will be raised if the cause is due to the heart, but commonly it is due to a hepatic vein thrombosis and therefore the pressure is very difficult to measure. Distinction between these three groups can be made on the basis of hepatic venography with hepatic vein wedged pressure measurement.

Causes of portal hypertension include:

1. Pre-sinusoidal / Extrahepatic obstruction:

   Extra hepatic causes include -
   Portal vein thrombosis (idiopathic, umbilical and portal sepsis, malignancy, hypercoagulable states, pancreatitis)
   Splenic vein thrombosis
   Sarcoid
   Myeloproliferative disease
   Intrahepatic causes include primary biliary cirrhosis, sclerosing cholangitis, Shistosomiasis

2. Sinusoidal / Hepatic causes

   Arsenic, vinyl chloride
   Fibropolycystic disease
   Cirrhosis of any cause eg chronic active hepatitis, alcoholic hepatitis
   Partial nodular transformation

3. Hepatic venous outflow obstruction

   Suprahepatic

   Budd-Chiari syndrome (vena cava web, hepatic vein thrombosis)
   Constrictive pericarditis
   Right heart failure

   Smaller hepatic veins and venules

   Veno-occlusive disease (eg. Antileukaemic drugs, radiation, Bush tea)
   Sclerosing hyaline necrosis

Beta-thalassaemia will cause iron overload if treated with transfusion which may cause secondary haemochromatosis, with hepatic fibrosis and hepatocellular failure.

Schistosoma mansoni and japonicum cause hepatosplenic disease due to progressive deposition of the eggs in the liver and intestinal tract. Schistosoma haematobium live in the venules draining the bladders and ureters and tend to cause genitourinary disease.

Hepatitis A does not cause chronic liver disease.

McIntyre N, Burroughs AK. Cirrhosis, portal hypertension and ascites. In Weatherall DJ, Ledingham JGG, Warrell DA, eds. Oxford Textbook of Medicine, Oxford: Oxford University Press, 1996.

Question 49

A. false **B.** true **C.** true **D.** true **E.** false

Paper 1 Question 48 lists the features of coeliac disease, which affects the whole of the small bowel: involvement of only the distal end is not characteristic. The presence of endomysial antibodies, delayed puberty and mouth ulcers are all features. Pyoderma gangrenosum is a feature of inflammatory bowel disease.

Coeliac disease in focus:

Coeliac disease principally affects caucasians, and to a lesser extent Indians and Arabs. It has a variable presentation from the asymptomatic individual picked up on screening to severe disease. There is an HLA association – HLA DQ2 (95%), HLA DQ8 (5%). DQ2 exists in cist and trans forms thus explaining the associations with HLA B8 & DR3. As a reflection of the HLA association, coeliac disease is seen in about 10% of first-degree relatives and there is a 70% concordance in identical twins. There is a variable prevalence in Europe 1:300 – 1:1,500.

The presentation of the disease has already been highlighted in Paper 1 Question 48:

1. In infants – classically soon after weaning at the point of introducing cereals

   babies fail to thrive, refuse to eat and lose weight. There may be abdominal distension, muscle wasting +/– diarrhoea. Abdominal pain may be prominent and mislead the physician. Rectal prolapse may be a feature.

2. In older children the presentation may include nutritional deficiencies, growth retardation and anaemias.

3. In adults the presentation may consist of anaemia (Fe & folate deficiency, low normal or high MCV), abdominal discomfort (bloating, excess wind and altered bowel habit), mouth ulcers, infertility in males/females. The irritable bowel syndrome (IBS) is a frequent mis-diagnosis. The classical description of a patient with features of malabsorption and malnutrition, including steatorrhoea, weight loss, weakness and bruising is now uncommon.

Associations: IDDM (5%), autoimmune thyroid disease, Addison's disease, pernicious anaemia, fibrosing alveolitis, SLE, polyarthritis, IgA deficiency (5%), Down's syndrome (5%), primary biliary cirrhosis, hyposplenism.

Diagnosis of coeliac disease: serum antibodies to gliaden (IgA isotype), IgA antibodies to reticulin (IgA endomysial antibodies) and antibodies to tissue transglutaminase which is now recognised as the autoantigen in coeliac disease. Serum autoantibodies have a false negative rate of 3–5% and therefore the gold standard is still considered to be a small intestinal biopsy. The currently recommended serological tests are total IgA level, IgA and IgG antigliadin antibodies and either antiendomysial or tissue transglutaminase antibodies.

Treatment of coeliac disease consists primarily of a gluten free diet (avoiding wheat, barley and rye). Oats is controversial but could be considered if the patient fails to improve. The management also includes: repeat histology at 6 months, patient education, advice on diet, dietician, referral to local coeliac society, vitamin replacement in the short term, looking for, and treatment of, osteoporosis. Iron and vitamin B_{12} replacement may be needed indefinitely in some patients, despite strict adherence to the diet and histological improvement

Schuppan D. Current concepts of coeliac disease pathogenesis Gastroenterology 2000 119: 234–242

Question 50

A. true **B.** true **C.** true **D.** true **E.** true

Oesophagitis is an endoscopic diagnosis where inflammation is manifested for example in ulceration or breaks in the mucosal membranes. A normal endoscopy does not exclude the diagnosis of acid/bile reflux as patients may still clearly experience pain in the absence of ulceration/inflammation. In systemic sclerosis fibrous connective tissue replaces smooth muscle in the GI tract affecting motility of the oesophagus (in 80% of cases) and the small bowel. Surgery is particularly hazardous in these patients. Radiological investigations of the small bowel may show fluid levels on AXR, flocculated barium on small bowel series and reduced motility and transit time. The full range of oesophageal abnormalities in these patients includes loss of peristalsis (70%), reflux (60%), dilatation (50%), absent lower oesophageal sphincter tone (40%), hiatus hernia (20%) and stricture (10%).

Gastrointestinal presentations of scleroderma:

1. reflux oesophagitis leading to regurgitation, epigastric pain or dysphagia

2. post prandial bloating secondary to gastric dilatation and delayed emptying or malabsortion
3. steatorrhoea from bacterial overgrowth (due to small intestinal hypomotility), lymphatic fibrosis
4. anaemia due to severe oesophagitis (plus or minus peptic ulceration), telangiectasia; bacterial overgrowth
5. constipation due to chronic intestinal pseudoobstruction, faecal impaction and iatrogenic (barium impaction)

Oesophageal strictures are a common complication of gastro-oesophageal reflux disease (GORD).

The symptoms of ischaemic heart disease can be difficult to differentiate from oesophageal reflux. Sublingual glyceryl trinitrate can improve the symptoms of GORD, causing further confusion though the temporal relationship between administration and pain relief may be worth exploring: for ischaemic heart disease pain relief within 5 minutes in stable angina is typical. The mechanism of action in relief of GORD may be due to reduction in oesophageal spasm. There has been much debate in the literature surrounding the issue of the relationship between asthma and GORD. There are several pathophysiologic mechanisms by which acid reflux can cause bronchospasm. In fact antireflux therapy in patients with asthma and GORD results in improvements in asthma outcome in as many as 70% to 80% of patients treated in both medical and surgical series. The role of acid and duodeno-gastro-oesophageal reflux (DGOR) or bile reflux is also controversial. DGOR alone is not injurious to oesophageal mucosa, but can result in significant esophageal mucosal injury when combined with acid reflux. Controlling oesophageal exposure to acid reflux by using proton pump inhibitors probably also eliminates the potentially damaging effect of GORD.

Kahrilas PJ. Gastroesophageal reflux disease.
JAMA 1996 276(12): 983–988

Richter JE. Gastroesophageal reflux disease and asthma: the two are directly related. American Journal of Medicine 2000 108 Suppl 4a: 153S–158S.

Vaezi MF, Richter JE. Importance of duodeno-gastro-esophageal reflux in the medical outpatient practice. Hepato-Gastroenterology 1999 46(25): 40–47.

Question 51

A. false **B.** false **C.** true **D.** true **E.** true

Protein losing enteropathy is a syndrome rather than a disease. It is the intestinal equivalent of nephrotic syndrome. Some causes are obvious exudative conditions like Crohn's disease or TB but others are subtle and may present as a mild hypoproteinaemia with no intestinal symptoms. It should be suspected in any patient who has hypoalbuminaemia in the absence of proteinuria, anorexia or an acute phase response to intercurrent illness. The diagnosis can be obtained with measurement of faecal chromium or faecal clearance of alpha 1 antitrypsin. Features include ascites, peripheral oedema, pleural effusions, marked hypoalbuminaemia in the absence of liver or renal disease, steatorrhoea and hypogammaglobulinaemia. Some causes:

Neoplastic: Kaposis sarcoma, neoplastic small bowel and abdominal lymphatic system disorders

Infection: dysentery, paracoccidiodomycosis, strongyloidiasis, schistosomiasis, trematodiasis, giardiasis, measles, small bowel bacterial overgrowth, tropical sprue

Inflammatory: Whipple's disease, Crohn's disease, congenital malformation of the small bowel and abdominal lymphatic system, connective tissue disorders, systemic lupus erythematosis, rheumatoid arthritis, systemic sclerosis with pancreatic insufficiency, Behçets disease, coeliac disease

Cardiac causes: cardiac cachexia, high venous pressure from congestive cardiac failure and constrictive pericarditis

Erythroderma: eczema, psoriasis, lymphoma

Other causes: intestinal lymphangiectasia, Menetrier's disease (giant hypertrophic gastritis), allergic gastroenteropathies.

Although hyperthyroidism can cause diarrhoea, there are no reports of resulting protein-losing enteropathy.

Jewell DP. Miscellaneous disorders of the gastrointestinal tract and liver. In Weatherall DJ, Ledingham JGG, Warrell DA, eds. Oxford Textbook of Medicine, Oxford: Oxford University Press, 1996.

Question 52

A. false **B.** true **C.** false **D.** false **E.** false

Causes of high T4/T3 and raised TSH/or non-suppressed TSH are given in the answer to Paper 2 Question 54.

Question 53

A. false **B.** false **C.** true **D.** false **E.** true

Diagnostic significance of tumour markers in serum.

Alpha-feto protein (AFP)

non-seminomatous germ-cell tumours (80%)
hepatocellular carcinoma (50%; i.e. up to 50% of HCC have a normal alpha fetoprotein; it is therefore too insensitive for screening)

Beta human chorionic gonadotrophin (HCG)

choriocarcinoma (100%)
non-seminomatous germ-cell tumours (50%)
seminoma (10%; elevation is generally mild)

Carcino-embryonic antigen (CEA)

colorectal cancer, especially if there are liver metastases, but poor sensitivity for early-stage disease; it is often elevated in advanced-stage gastric, breast and lung cancer; not used for screening but may be useful for follow-up; may help in distinguishing undifferentiated carcinoma (if positive) from poorly differentiated lymphoma or melanoma

Prostate-specific antigen (PSA)

elevated in 95% of primary prostate cancers
levels reflect degree of extra-prostatic extension
if elevated in asymptomatic patients may indicate the need for transrectal ultrasound and/or needle biopsy

Prostatic acid phosphatase (PAP)

prostatic carcinoma, esp. bone secondaries (85% positive)
poor sensitivity for early-stage disease (50% false negative)
less sensitive monitor of tumour activity than PSA, and elevations of either occur in benign prostatic hypertrophy

Calcitonin

used in medullary carcinoma of the thyroid for screening, diagnosis and follow-up

Alkaline phosphatase

elevation may signify metastasis to bone or liver. In bone disease the enzyme is heat-labile, and there is no elevation of gamma-GT

Thyroglobulin [not thyroxine-binding globulin!]

papillary/follicular thyroid cancer
used in follow-up

Ca 125

ovarian cancer, especially non-mucinous.
positive in 80% of cases. Predicts recurrence in 75%
not specific for ovarian ca. Also positive in endometrial carcinoma with peritoneal seedlings

Ca15–3

breast cancer
positive in 75% of cases with metastases

Ca 19–9

gastrointestinal cancer, especially pancreas or biliary

Epstein RJ. Medicine for examinations. 3rd Ed. Churchill Livingstone, London, 1996.

Question 54

A. false **B.** true **C.** true **D.** false **E.** true

Thyrotoxicosis is a rare disorder of childhood that is characterized by an accelerated metabolism of body tissues, which results from the stimulation of thyroid gland activity induced through a variety of autoantibodies. Historically less than 5% of all incidents of Graves' disease occur in childhood, and recent studies show an incidence as low as 1 per million. It is three to eight times more prevalent in females than in males and increases in incidence throughout childhood and adolescence. More than two thirds of childhood cases occur between the ages of 10 and 15 years. Thyrotoxicosis increases skeletal growth before skeletal maturity; there is increased activity of both forming and resorbing cells, although the imbalance is in favour of resorption.

Turner's syndrome is a common (1 in 2500) disorder, with a 45X karyotype; complete absence of one X chromosome, although some mosaics have typical features. Generally it presents in either infancy or childhood. Short stature may be the only significant feature, and a large number of affected girls have only subtle clinical signs. Puberty is usually, but not always absent. Also associated are aortic coarctation, webbing of the neck, cubitus valgus, hirsutism and peripheral oedema. Intelligence is normal.

Childhood Crohn's disease can cause short stature, and in fact often presents as failure to thrive, or with delayed puberty with no gastrointestinal symptoms. Malnutrition and vitamin deficiencies are common.

Isolated gonadotrophin deficiency in most instances results from GnRH deficiency, although any of the gonadotrophins may be involved. This tends to cause delayed onset of puberty, but growth hormones are not affected so generally growth until that point is normal. It is often not until puberty fails to occur that suspicion is aroused.

Achondroplasia causes a striking disproportion between the trunk that is of normal length and the short arms and legs with a large skull. The fingertips may only reach the iliac crest. There is lumbar lordosis, wedging of the upper lumbar vertebrae and occasionally this develops into a lumbar lordosis. These children are intellectually normal. Homozygous achondroplasia is lethal. Hypochondroplasia is inherited independently from achondroplasia, with an unaffected skull, and less skeletal disproportion and fewer spinal abnormalities, although still with relatively short stature.

Gregory JW. The short child: clinical assessment and treatment. British Journal of Hospital Medicine 1994 52(7): 339–341

Question 55

A. true **B.** true **C.** false **D.** false **E.** false

Diabetes mellitus is an enormous subject, expect to have to answer questions on it in all aspects of the exam from MCQs in Part I to short cases and long cases in part II. There is a great deal of information in both the OTM and Harrisons, the principal reference books.

It is clear that there is a substantial genetic component to type I diabetes. The disease runs in families, with siblings having a 6% risk of developing the disease vs. 0.4% of the normal population, although the pattern is complex, and it is likely that multiple gene loci are involved. The two loci that have been implicated, HLA and insulin (INS) are said to account for only 30% of total genetic susceptibility. HLA was originally implicated in diabetes susceptibility with HLA B8 and B15. HLA DR3 and DR4 give increased susceptibility as do DR1, DR8 and DR5. Disease protection is provided by DR2. Twin studies suggest that only 30% of the disease susceptibility is genetic in IDDM, although some twin studies in type 2 diabetes suggest as high as 90% concordance.

Most IDDM patients have circulating autoantibodies to beta cell antigens, including insulin and glutamic acid decarboxylase, as well as anti-islet-cell antibodies.

Type 1 patients do not have microvascular disease at presentation, as these changes are generally related to chronicity of disease, and it is unlikely that at presentation these patients have had the disease for years. Type 2 patients often have microvascular changes on presentation, as they have often had the disease for many years (even 10 or 20) before diagnosis.

Type 1 patients produce no insulin, hence the phrase insulin-dependent, so do not have high post-prandial insulin levels. Type 2 diabetic patients do often have high insulin levels, particularly post-prandial, as insulin-resistance often plays an important part in the pathophysiology of the disease.

Bell JI, Hockaday TDR. Diabetes Mellitus. In Weatherall DJ, Ledingham JGG, Warrell DA, eds. Oxford Textbook of Medicine, Oxford: Oxford University Press, 1996.

Question 56

A. true **B.** false **C.** true **D.** false **E.** true

Erythema nodosum is an acute panniculitis causing painful nodule or plaques on the skin. In certain cases it may be recurrent. It is associated with malaise, fever and arthralgia. It slowly fades leaving bruises and staining of the skin. In around 50% no cause is found. The differential includes:

pregnancy
oral contraceptive pill
post streptococcal infections
inflammatory bowel disease
sarcoidosis
leprosy
yersinia
TB
malignancy
sulphonamides
chlamydia

Jones SK. Skin manifestations of systemic disease
Medicine 2000 28:11; 34–37

Question 57

A. true **B.** true **C.** false **D.** false **E.** false

Proximal (type II) renal tubular acidosis results from an inability to reabsorb bicarbonate in the proximal tubule which results in marked renal bicarbonate wasting and the development of a hyperchloraemic hypokalaemic metabolic acidosis with a normal anion gap. The lowered bicarbonate threshold means the plasma bicarbonate level decreases until a steady state is reached at which stage the kidney can again appropriately acidify the urine due to a reduced level of filtered bicarbonate. The ability to acidify the urine in the presence of severe systemic acidosis helps differentiate proximal from distal RTA. Proximal renal tubular acidosis is usually associated with more general tubular abnormalities such as glycosuria, aminoaciduria, hyperphosphaturia, and uricosuria as part of the Fanconi syndrome. Familial cases are rare and generally present in infancy with failure to thrive and polyuria. Nephrocalcinosis and renal calculi do not occur though there is an association with rickets and osteomalacia due to renal phosphate losses. Treatment is with oral bicarbonate and extremely high doses may be required to overcome the renal leak. Hypokalaemia persists and potassium supplements are usually necessary.

Type IV renal tubular acidosis presents with a hyperkalaemic hyperchloraemic normal anion gap acidosis. This is generally in response to hypoaldosteronism either secondary to Addison's disease or due to low renin production as seen in diabetes and chronic tubulointerstitial disease or secondary to NSAID use. Mineralocorticoid should be used for treatment if the acidosis is severe.

Causes of proximal RTA include Cystinosis, Wilson's disease, hereditary fructose intolerance, multiple myeloma, lead poisoning, outdated tetracycline therapy, hyperparathyroidism, and the nephrotic syndrome.

Unwin RJ, Capasso G. The Renal Tudular Acidoses
J R Soc Med 2001 94: 221–225

Question 58

A. false **B.** true **C.** true **D.** true **E.** true

The glomerular injury that occurs in immune-complex nephritis is the result of both humoral and cell-mediated immunity. There are three basic mechanisms by which antigen-antibody complexes may lead to the development of glomerulonephritis.

1. Antibodies may form that are directed against a structural component of the glomerulus. Eg. anti-glomerular basement membrane antibody in Goodpasture's syndrome.
2. Antigens may be deposited (planted) in the glomerulus in certain disease states which then act as targets for antibodies to complex with. Eg Histone-DNA complexes in SLE which are targeted by anti-DNA antibodies.
3. Pre-formed circulating antigen-antibody complexes may be filtered and deposited in the glomerulus. Eg. Post-streptococcal glomerulonephritis.

The area of the glomerulus involved is dependent on the molecular size and charge of the antigen or complexes involved. Highly cationic particles cross the glomerular basement membrane and are deposited in subepithelial locations while highly anionic particles cannot cross the glomerular basement membrane and are trapped subendothelially. Neutrally charged molecules tend to be deposited in the mesangium. The pattern of involvement is also affected by changes in mesangial function, the integrity of the glomerular basement membrane, and changes in glomerular blood flow. This gives rise to the various histological pictures seen with immune-complex nephritis dependent on which glomerular structures are involved.

Histological localization of immune complexes in glomerulonephritis

Subepithelial humps e.g. acute glomerulonephritis

Epimembranous deposits e.g. membranous glomerulonephritis

Subendothelial deposits e.g. SLE and membranoproliferative glomerulonephritis

Mesangial deposits e.g. IgA nephropathy

The collecting ducts are not involved in glomerulonephritis.

Cotran RS, Kumar V, Collins T (Eds). Robbins Pathological Basis of Disease 6th Ed. 1999 W.B. Saunders Philadelphia.

Question 59

A. false **B.** false **C.** true **D.** true **E.** true

Minimal change glomerulonephritis accounts for 25% of cases of adult nephrotic syndrome and over 80% of cases in children under the age of eight. It is associated with Hodgkins lymphoma, carcinoma, atopy, and NSAID use though most cases are idiopathic. There is an association with HLA-DR7 in Europe and HLA-DR8 in Japan.

Glomeruli appear normal on light microscopy though on electron microscopy there is effacement of the podocyte foot processes and a minor degree of mesangial IgM deposits and mesangial proliferation in some cases. On presentation 30% of adults are hypertensive, 30% have microscopic haematuria, and 60% have a degree of renal impairment. These findings are all rare in children. Renal biopsy is essential in adults presenting with the nephrotic syndrome.

Treatment: 80% respond to oral steroids though prolonged courses may be necessary. Patients with multiple relapses may require cyclophosphamide or cyclosporin. Progression of steroid responsive disease to endstage renal failure is rare.

Adu D. Idiopathic Glomerulonephritis.
Oxford Textbook of Medicine. Oxford University Press.

Question 60

A. true **B.** true **C.** false **D.** false **E.** false

Urinary calculi are a common problem worldwide with calcium containing stones predominating in developed countries. Predisposing factors include dehydration, diet, urinary composition, pH, urinary stasis, and infection. In the UK calcium oxalate stones make up 66% of cases, triple-phosphate (infection) stones 15%, uric acid stones 6%, cystine stones 3%, and others the rest.

Calcium stones are often recurrent and may be familial with hypercalciuria being demonstrable in the majority of cases. Hyperuricosuria and hyperoxaluria both also contribute to the formation of calcium oxalate stones. In cases of fat malabsorption (e.g. small bowel resection) the excess free fatty acids in the bowel bind to calcium which leaves oxalate unbound and free to be absorbed from the colon producing urinary hyperoxaluria. This leads to the formation of urinary stones and in rare cases renal failure.

Triple-phosphate stones generally occur in alkaline infected urine, in contrast to other stones, and are commoner in women. Proteus, in particular, cleaves urea forming ammonia which raises the urinary pH predisposing to stone formation.

Cystinuria is an autosomal recessive inborn error of dibasic amino acid metabolism with an incidence of 1:7000 live births. It predisposes to the development of radio-opaque cystine stones which typically present with pain and haematuria.

Treatment

Calcium stones – oral phosphate and high fluid intake

Phosphate stones – eradicate infection

Uric acid stones – alkalinization of urine or allopurinol

Cystine stones – alkalinization of urine and high fluid intake +/- penicillamine

Keen CE. Urinary Calculi
Medicine 1999 27 (7): 93–95

Paper 4 Answers

Question 1

A. true **B.** false **C.** false **D.** true **E.** false

Chromosomes are usually visualized during mitosis, at metaphase. At this stage the DNA is coiled and condensed, and the chromosomes consist of two identical chromatids, joined together at the centromere. The position of the centromere is specific for each chromosome: in some it is close to the centre (metacentric) whilst in others it is near one end (acrocentric). All chromosomes are divided by the centromere into a short arm (p) and a long arm (q). Abnormalities in chromosomes relate either to their number or to structural problems (breakage or rearrangement).

The normal diploid number of chromosomes in humans is 46. Individuals with counts that are not multiples of the normal haploid number (23) are said to be aneuploid. A fetus can have multiples of 23 e.g. 69 or 92 chromosomes: such triploid or tetraploid fetuses will miscarry quite early. Individuals with one extra chromosome are trisomic for that particular chromosome. Two extra chromosomes is termed double trisomy. Monosomy arises where one chromosome is missing. It is rare to get monosomy in live children except in the X chromosomes giving monosomy X (Turner's syndrome). Structural changes in chromosomes:

Deletion: breakage of chromosomes resulting in loss of material

Reciprocal translocation: exchange of information between two non-identical chromosomes

Inversion of a segment of chromosome can either involve the centromere (pericentric inversion) or on the short or long arms eg long arm of the X chromosome as in Haemophilia A

Ring chromosome – two ends of one chromosome join together

Robertsonian translocation involves the translocation between the long arms of two acrocentric chromosomes joined at the centromere

See question Paper 3 Question 1 for a list of abnormal karyotypes. Examples of karyotype nomenclature:

46, XX	normal female
45, X	Turner's syndrome
47, XY +21	male with trisomy 21
69 XXY	triploidy, XXY sex chromosome complement
45, X/46, XX	mosaic Turner's syndrome

46, XX, t(9:21)(q11:p11) means that chromosome 9 has broken at band q11 and chromosome 21 has broken at band p11. 't' signifies translocation: material has been exchanged between the two chromosomes.

A translocation between chromosomes 8 and 14 (t[8;14][q24.13: q32.33]) is characteristic of Burkitt's lymphoma. The abnormalities involving chromosome 14 have been found in relation to a variety of other lymphomas, particularly of B-cell origin. CGL has a distinct chromosome marker, the Ph chromosome, resulting from the reciprocal translocation t(9;22), which is found in 95 per cent of cases.

Pembrey ME. Genetic factors in disease
Oxford Textbook of Medicine. Oxford University Press.

Question 2

A. false **B.** true **C.** true **D.** false **E.** false

Until recently Marfan's syndrome was considered a problem of collagen but it is now recognized that it is caused by mutations in the epidermal growth factor-like regions of the fibrillin gene on chromosome 15. Fibrillin is the major constituent of the microfibrillar system and of the suspensory ligament of the lens – hence the association between aortic dissection and dislocation of the lens. Whilst not all patients suffer from a dissection most will get aortic dilatation – usually at the proximal part of the sinus of Valsalva and returning to normal below the innominate artery. The cusps of the aortic valve do not close properly. If a dissection occurs it usually begins in the area of greatest dilatation and may progress proximally or distally. Retrograde dissection may tear the attachment of the coronary arteries and rupture into the pericardial sac.

Marfan's syndrome is dominantly inherited. Whilst the major effects are in the skeletal, cardiovascular and ocular systems, there is wide variation phenotypically. In the classical patient the following are recognized:

tall stature
limbs long relative to the trunk
arachnodactyly
hypermobility
scoliosis
narrow and high arched or "Gothic" palate

eye problems: dislocation of the lens (usually upwards and temporally)
reduced vision / myopia
squint
iris trembles with small eye movements (iridodonesis) because it is poorly supported by an abnormally mobile lens
retinal detachments
glaucoma

aortic incompetence and dissection
colonic diverticulae
mitral valve prolapse
tricuspid valve prolapse
phenotype similar to homocystinuria

Less well known features:

dural ectasia
spontaneous pneumothorax: the occurrence of bullous emphysematous changes in lung apices can lead to pneumothorax in 5% of cases
cutaneous striae / recurrent purpura or skin bruising
impaired platelet adhesion
herniae

Diagnosis will probably be easier in the future with the isolated gene defect. Classically it rests on: family history, exclusion of homocystinuria and phenotypic presentation. Treatment is aimed at monitoring the aortic valve and aorta with a view to surgery, β-blockers to reduce left ventricular systole, correction of myopia, correction of scoliosis, prophylactic antibiotics for procedures and genetic counselling.

Causes of mitral valve prolapse:

Idiopathic
Pseudoxanthoma elasticum
Ehlers Danlos
Osteogenesis imperfecta
Marfan's syndrome

Smith R. Disorders of the skeleton
Oxford Textbook of Medicine. Oxford University Press.

Question 3

A. false **B.** true **C.** true **D.** true **E.** false

Complement receptor Type I (CRI) is present on peripheral B lymphocytes, erythrocytes, monocytes and tissue macrophages. Chemokines are a group of small, cysteine-rich proteins with strong sequence homology between members that include the following:

Interleukin 8 (IL-8)

Monocyte chemotactic peptide (MCP)

Macrophage inflammatory proteins 1alpha and 1beta

Each is a specific chemoattractant for different groups of leucocytes. For instance, IL-8 is a specific chemoattractant for neutrophils, while MCP attracts predominantly monocytes.

Keshav S. Cytokines
Oxford Textbook of Medicine. Oxford University Press.

Question 4

A. false **B.** false **C.** true **D.** true **E.** true

Continuous basal secretion of nitric oxide (NO) is responsible for endothelium dependent dilator tone. It is a potent vasodilator, synthesized from L-arginine and has a half-life of only a few seconds. On secretion it diffuses from the endothelium into the underlying smooth muscle where it binds to the haem moiety of guanylate cyclase. The subsequent increase in cyclic guanosine monophosphate relaxes the smooth muscle. At the luminal surface NO also inhibits platelet activation. The physiological upregulators for NO may include shear stress and platelet-derived mediators such as acetylcholine, bradykinin and substance P. In veins there does not appear to be the same basal secretion however vasodilatation does occur on NO release. (NO is the active moiety of glyceryl trinitrate – hence the therapeutic advantage in, for example, heart failure).

NO together with prostacyclin (PGE2) are two important inhibitors of platelet aggregation. Both may also inhibit the adhesion of white cells to endothelium. A number of cytokines and drugs increase the synthesis or release of NO:

Interleukin I
Tumour necrosis factor
ACE inhibitor (by inhibition of bradykinin)

Vallance P. Vascular endothelium, its physiology and pathophysiology. Oxford Textbook of Medicine. Oxford University Press.

Question 5

A. true **B.** true **C.** false **D.** true **E.** false

Muscles supplied by the median nerve include:

1. lateral two lumbricals
2. opponens pollicis
3. abductor pollicis brevis
4. flexor pollicis brevis

Causes of wasting of the small muscles of the hand

1. disuse	old age rheumatoid arthritis
2. spinal cord lesion	syringomyelia motor neurone disease
3. spinal cord compression	cervical spondylosis C8 / T1 tumour
4. bilateral nerve root compression	cervical spondylosis thoracic outlet syndrome
5. peripheral neuropathy	Charcot Marie Tooth disease lead poisoning acute intermittent porphyria

Testing the nerve root integrity of the upper limb

1. C5: shoulder abduction (deltoid)

   "Make wings with your elbows, keep them up, don't let me push them down"
2. C5/C6: elbow flexion (biceps)

   "pull me towards you"
3. C7: elbow extension (triceps)

   "now push me away"
4. C8: finger flexion long and short finger flexors

   "squeeze my fingers hard"

5. T1: finger abduction / adduction (intrinsic hand muscles) "spread you fingers apart, dont let me push them in"

Ger R, Abrahams P. Essentials of Clinical Anatomy
London Pitman Publishing

Question 6

A. false **B.** false **C.** true **D.** false **E.** true

Brown Sequard syndrome may be caused by compression or inflammatory disease of the spinal cord and occasionally with vascular lesions. Other lesions include mass fractures of the vertebrae or penetrating injuries. Signs of hemisection of the cord:

1. there is ipsilateral sensory loss over one or several segments at the level of the lesion (D1 would therefore affect medial aspect of the right arm in T1 dermatome
2. ipsilateral dorsal column sensory impairment
3. ipsilateral pyramidal signs
4. contralateral spinothalamic sensory impairment (pain and temperature)

To summarize: spastic weakness on the side of the lesion, loss of pain and thermal sensation contralateral side and light touch is intact.

Causes of acute / subacute paraplegia

1.	trauma	
2.	vertebral diseases	metastatic carcinoma cervical spondylosis Paget's disease rheumatoid arthritis
3.	tumour	extradural / intradural carcinoma e.g. lymphoma, myeloma, leukaemia, neurofibroma
4.	haematological	all cases of thrombocytopenia other clotting diseases leukaemia over anticoagulation
5.	infection	epidural abscess TB abscess

		syphilitic myelitis HIV infection vascular myelopathy
6.	vascular	anterior spinal artery occlusion infarction e.g. secondary to hypotension, emboli or aortic dissection vasculitis
7.	inflammatory	myelitis multiple sclerosis SLE sarcoidosis
8.	metabolic	subacute degeneration of the cord

Scadding JW, Gibby J. Neurological disease
Oxford Textbook of Medicine. Oxford University Press.

Question 7

A. true **B.** false **C.** true **D.** false **E.** false

Vasovagal syndrome or the common faint is one of the differentials for syncope. The upright posture is an invariable feature leading to the pooling of 500 to 1000ml of blood in the lower limbs and to reduction in central blood volume. Levels of Adrenaline and vasopressin appear to be elevated above normal prior to the attack causing increased left ventricular contraction and sensitization of the left ventricular baroreceptors. There may be tachycardia and hypertension prior to the episode. On standing there is reduced cardiac filling that triggers the sensitized baroreceptors leading to bradycardia and vasodilatation. In the context of pre-existing low central blood volume this is an unstable situation for maintaining blood pressure and on many occasions the fall in blood pressure leads to unconsciousness and collapse to the ground. Vasovagal syncope has never been documented to occur in bed and rarely in the horizontal position. Typical circumstances for the episode to occur include crowded trains, waiting at bus stops or in school assembly.

Causes of syncope:

Common faint	***prolonged standing***
Postural hypotension	elderly drugs orthostatic hypotension

Valsalva mechanism	playing wind instruments
Micturition syncope	
Cough syncope	
Carotid sinus disease	
Cardiac syncope	sick sinus syndrome
Arrhythmias	tachyarrhythmias, bradyarrhythmias
Structural	HOCM
	valvular stenosis
	constrictive pericarditis
	atrial myxoma
Hypovolaemia	haemorrhage
	Addison's disease
Autonomic (areflexic)	
	diabetes
	polyneuropathy
	tabes dorsalis
	Shy-Drager syndrome
	drugs
	quadriplegia
Metabolic	hypoxia
	hypoglycaemia
Hyperventilation	
Vertigo	vestibular disease

Blumhardt LD. Syncope
Oxford Textbook of Medicine. Oxford University Press.

Question 8

A. false **B.** true **C.** true **D.** true **E.** false

Effects and clinical features of hypoglycaemia

Autonomic:	Increased sympathetic activation	tremor
		sweating
		tachycardia
	Neuroglycopenia	hunger
		confusion
		abnormal behaviour
		fitting
		coma

Symptoms may be non-specific and hypoglycaemia may remain unrecognized for years: recurrent or chronic hypoglycaemia has caused people to be institutionalized for suspected psychiatric disease. Hypoglycaemia is defined as a blood glucose level of < 2.2 mmol/l. Causes of hypoglycaemia:

Exogenous administration e.g. by medical staff	
Insulinoma	
Addison's disease	
Pituitary failure	
Drugs	insulin sulphonylureas pentamidine ethanol salicylate overdose (in children)
Hepatic disorders	acute liver failure glycogen storage disease
Hereditary fructose intolerance	
Post gastric surgery	(reactive hypoglycaemia)
Miscellaneous:	malnutrition prolonged exercise falciparum malaria autoimmune (antibodies to the active insulin receptor)

Wilding J, Williams G. Diabetes Mellitus and disorders of lipid and intermediary metabolism. Medicine Souhami/Moxham Churchill Livingston

Question 9

A. false **B.** true **C.** false **D.** true **E.** false

Actions of angiotensin II:

1. potent vasoconstrictor
2. stimulates release of aldosterone (and therefore sodium retention)
3. reduces renin release from kidney (homeostatic mechanism) and therefore reduces intraglomerular pressure
4. expression of proto-oncogenes; cell growth
5. promotes microalbuminuria
6. increases plasminogen activator leading to impaired fibrinolysis

Opie LH. Drugs for the heart
Saunders. Philadelphia

Question 10

A. false **B.** true **C.** true **D.** false **E.** false

Effect of hypothermia:

Increased catecholamine drive to the heart
Ventricular fibrillation (secondary to catecholamine release)
Frost bite
Acute pancreatitis
Transient thrombocytopenia
Hypoglycaemia
Metabolic acidosis
Potassium accumulation in the extracellular space
Bradycardia
Confusion, stupor, coma
Shallow respiration
Hypotension
Oedema of face and eyelids
Normal tendon reflexes (unless hypothyroidism)

ECG changes: bradycardia
J waves
atrial fibrillation
slow ventricular response

Causes of sinus bradycardia:

Physiological: sleep
young people
athletes

Sinoatrial disease

Drugs: beta blockers
amiodarone
calcium channel blockers

Vagotonia vasovagal syndrome
inferior myocardial infarction

Hypothyroidism
Hypothermia
Jaundice
Raised intracranial pressure

Ward FI, Evans JG. Medicine in old age
Oxford Textbook of Medicine. Oxford University Press.

Question 11

A. true **B.** false **C.** false **D.** false **E.** true

Common causes of hypercalcaemia:

1. hyperparathyroidism
2. malignancy

Steroid suppressible:

3. sarcoidosis
4. vitamin D intoxication
5. multiple myeloma

Other causes:

immobilization
phaeochromocytoma (part of MEN type II)
artefact: venous stasis, hyperalbuminaemia (dehydration, parenteral nutrition), hypergammaglobulinaemia (myeloma, sarcoid)
milk alkali syndrome
thyrotoxicosis
thiazide diuretics
adrenal failure
familial hypocalciuric hypercalcaemia
haemodialysis
vitamin A
acute renal failure
VIPoma

Causes of hypocalcaemia:

hypoparathyroidism
osteomalacia / rickets
chronic renal failure
rare causes include low magnesium (inhibits PTH secretion)
pseudohypoparathyroidism
acute pancreatitis
chemotherapy: tubular damage by cisplatin leading to hypomagnesaemia
drugs: calcitonin, phosphate, diphosphonates
low plasma albumin: malnutrition, liver disease etc

Kanis JA. Disorders of calcium metabolism
Oxford Textbook of Medicine. Oxford University Press.

Question 12

A. false **B.** true **C.** true **D.** true **E.** false

The basic structure of an immunoglobulin molecule (e.g. IgG) consists of two identical (L) and two identical (H) chains. The N-terminal domains of both L and H chains are highly variable: they contain the antigen binding sites. The constant domains of the heavy chains define the isotype of the antibody: IgG, A, D, M or E each of which has particular functions. The isotypes determine specific properties of the antibody e.g. binding of the C1q of the complement system, binding of the Fc receptor enabling antibody to cross the placenta and binding of Fc receptor on mast cell and basophils. Light chain constant regions are one of two classes kappa and lambda.

Delves PJ, Roitt IM. The Immune System I
NEJM 2000 343: 1; 37–49

Delves PJ, Roitt IM. The Immune System II
NEJM 2000 343: 2; 108–117

Question 13

A. false **B.** false **C.** false **D.** true **E.** true

Terminology in transplantation:

1. Autograft (autologous)
   Transplantation of self i.e. individuals own tissue to another site e.g. covering of third degree burns with skin from a preserved area
2. Isograft (isogenic)
   Transplantation between genetically identical members e.g. renal transplant between two monozygotic identical twins
3. Allograft (allogenic)
   Transplantation between non-identical members of same species e.g. cadaveric renal transplant
4. Xenograft (xenogenic)
   Transplantation of tissues between members of different species e.g. a baboon transplanted into a human

Cascalho M, Platt JL. The Immunological barrier to xenotransplantation
Immunity 2001 14: 4; 437–446 (Review)

Question 14

A. false **B.** false **C.** true **D.** false **E.** true

Lyme disease is caused by Borrelia burgdorferi (B. burgdorferi), a spirochaete. It is transmitted via ixodid ticks. Around 10,000 cases are reported annually in the USA and 500 cases annually in the United Kingdom. Infection can occur in any age group and is most likely in individuals whose residence, work or recreational activities take them to areas where ticks are prevalent. Ixodid ticks are common in woodland, heath and moorland but can occur in semi rural areas adjacent to large populations. They attach themselves to their hosts by barbed mouthparts and transmit the spirochaetes through infected saliva. Humans are not crucial to the life cycle and in fact the major reservoirs for the organisms reside in small and medium sized mammals and birds. Infection can be minimized by wearing appropriate clothing in high-risk areas particularly during the high season of tick bites (late spring to early autumn), and by removing any ticks noted to be attached to skin. The longer the tick is attached the higher the incidence of Lyme disease; for ticks feeding less than 24–36hrs infection is less likely to occur. B. burgdorferi spreads via the blood stream and lymphatics to distant sites and may penetrate the blood brain barrier. Evasion of the hosts immune response may occur by way of altering its outer surface proteins (OSP) from OspC in the early stages to OspA and OspB in established infection. Individuals with a certain genetic makeup may be predisposed to infection (especially those who are HLA-DR4 positive).

Although infection may be asymptomatic and individuals with untreated infection may not progress to experience all phases, the disease may be divided into three stages:

Stage I: Localized borreliosis

Most common stage

Often only the rash present (erythema migrans); occurs 2–30 days after a bite

The rash may be distinctive on occasion with a pronounced margin that spreads out radially and has a central area that becomes clear as the affected skin returns to normal.

Local lymphadenopathy

Stage II: Early disseminated borreliosis

Systemic spread of the infection (over months) principally affecting: nervous, musculoskeletal and cardiovascular systems.

Flu-like illness (myalgia, arthralgia)

Further rashes: multiple areas of erythema migrans can occur (uncommon)

Early neurological presentations include:

- isolated facial palsy (+/– bilateral)
- other cranial nerve lesions
- lymphocytic meningitis
- and painful radiculoneuritis.

Musculoskeletal complications:

- persistent arthralgia
- small joint arthritis
- Recurrent episodes of large joint inflammation (especially affecting the knee) that may continue despite antibiotic treatment.

Cardiac manifestations: conduction abnormalities (usually mild, uncommon) and cardiomyopathy (rare)

Other systems affected: ocular
hepatic

Stage III: Chronic borreliosis (uncommon)

In the USA the most common presentation is chronic Lyme arthritis; in a minority the inflammation may continue for years after treatment with antibiotics. Other manifestations include radiculoneuropathy (predominantly sensory), Lyme encephalopathy (uncommon), poor memory and concentration, and subtle learning difficulties.

Rarely, Lyme encephalomyelitis may occur, consisting of spastic paraparesis, cognitive impairment, cranial neuropathy, bladder dysfunction and dysarthria.

Acrodermatitis chronica atrophicans is a chronic skin manifestation which is a violaceous skin rash that may last for years, and eventually become atrophic.

Investigations:

1. Borrelia culture (slow, low yield)
2. PCR for Borrelia DNA in skin biopsy of erythema migrans
3. Borrelia antibody testing (needs to be interpreted in the clinical setting as may be falsely positive in patients with infectious mononucleosis, rheumatoid disease, autoimmune disease and other spirochaetal infections; may be falsely negative in early erythema migrans).

Treatment consists of prolonged courses (for tissue penetration) of penicillin or doxycycline.

O'Connell S. Lyme disease
Medicine 2001 29: 3; 96–98

Steere AC. Lyme disease
NEJM 2001; 345: 115–125

Question 15

A. false **B.** true **C.** true **D.** false **E.** false

Clostridium difficile is the cause of an antibiotic induced colitis. There are two toxins produced, A and B. Many antibiotics (including metronidazole) can cause it but the most frequently implicated are cephalosporins.

It usually starts within a few days of starting antibiotics but can occur some time after stopping treatment. It causes fever, diarrhoea and abdominal pain.

It affects the large bowel only. Sigmoidoscopy can reveal an inflamed, ulcerated mucosa covered by a thin membrane like material hence the term pseudomembranous colitis. Sigmoidoscopy may be normal so it is essential to test stool for the presence of the toxin if clinically suspicious. Treatment is with oral vancomycin or metronidazole.

Pathan N et al. Diarrhoea
Medicine 2001 29; 2; 49–53

Question 16

A. true **B.** true **C.** false **D.** true **E.** false

Plasmodium malariae, vivax, and ovale comprise the benign malarias. Whilst they can cause a severe febrile illness with splenomegaly and anaemia they are very rarely fatal. Splenic rupture is the most serious complication. The incubation period is 2–3 weeks for P. vivax and P. ovale, and 3–6 weeks for P. malariae. However P. vivax and P. ovale have a persistent hepatic cycle so relapses may occur months to years after leaving an endemic country. P. malariae does not have a hepatic stage but may relapse years later due to persistent low level previously undetectable parasitaemia.

The acute symptoms are of a paroxysmal febrile illness though the typical tertiary (48hr) and quaternary (72hr) fever of P. vivax / P. ovale and P. malariae respectively, rarely occurs. Treatment is usually with 3 days of oral chloroquine. Patients suffering from P. vivax or P. ovale should then receive a two week course of primaquine to eradicate the hepatic hypnozoites to prevent further relapse. Chloroquine resistance is now emerging in some strains of P. vivax though as the risk from the disease is low it still remains the first line treatment. Primaquine may precipitate acute haemolysis in G6PD deficiency so patients should have their status determined prior to commencing therapy.

Sickle cell trait confers a protective benefit in P. falciparum due to a lower degree of parasitaemia in affected individuals, thus reducing the risk of serious complications.

Molyneux M. Malaria in non-endemic areas
Medicine 1997 25(1): 28–31

Question 17

A. true **B.** false **C.** false **D.** true **E.** false

Epstein-Barr virus is the cause of infectious mononucleosis and has also been implicated in the development of Burkitts lymphoma, nasopharyngeal carcinoma, oral hairy leukoplakia, post transplant lymphoma, and lymphoma in AIDS patients.

EBV may also be associated with Hodgkin's lymphoma and some types of gastric carcinoma. Recent work has identified the presence of EBV DNA in Reed-Sternberg cells though as yet a causal relationship has not been confirmed.

For discussion on infectious mononucleosis see Paper 5 Question 14.

Question 18

A. false **B.** true **C.** false **D.** true **E.** false

Haemoglobin is made up of 4 protein subunits each linked to a haem group. Adult haemoglobin is made up of 2 alpha and 2 beta subunits. All globins related to alpha globin are located on chromosome 16; those related to beta globins are located on chromosome 11.

Fetal haemoglobin comprises 2 alpha and 2 gamma subunits. After birth the production of gamma globin decreases and delta and beta globins are produced. Adult haemoglobin is predominantly a2b2, with small amounts of HbF and a2d2. HbF binds oxygen more tightly.

Haemoglobin abnormalities fall into 2 major groups:

1. Structural

   These are due to alterations in the DNA coding leading to structural abnormal globin eg sickle cell anaemia.

2 Imbalanced Globin Chain Production

   Globins are structurally normal but the relative amounts are incorrect. This is the underlying problem in the thalassaemias. The thalassaemias are named after the affected gene, so that in alpha thalassaemia there is abnormality of production such that alpha globin is either reduced or abolished from red cells.

   Pre natal testing is available for sickle cell anaemia. It requires chorionic villous sampling in the 1st trimester or fetal blood sampling in the 2nd trimester. There are oligonucleotide probes which are specific for the point mutations in sickle cell anaemia.

Provan D, Chisholm M, Duncombe A, Singer C, Smith A
Oxford Handbook of Clinical Haematology Oxford University Press 1998

Question 19

A. false **B.** false **C.** false **D.** false **E.** true

Factor VIII and factor VIIa activate factor X to become factor Xa. It has a biological half-life of 8–12 hours. Factor VIII is part of the intrinsic pathway. Haemophilia A is a deficiency of VIII:C. It is inherited as an X linked recessive disorder. The severity of the disease is dependent on the level of the factorVII:C. If the level is less than 1% then there are frequent episodes of spontaneous bleeding in early life. There may be joint deformities as a consequence of recurrent haemarthroses. If the level is between 1–5% severe bleeding is usually only seen after an injury but they are prone to spontaneous epistaxis. At levels greater than 5% post traumatic bleeding is the only clinical abnormality usually. Recombinant factor VIII is now available. Previously it was extracted from human blood and unfortunately many haemophiliacs contracted HIV/HCV before screening for these viruses was introduced. It is associated with normal bleeding time and prothrombin time. The PTTK/APTT is prolonged.

In von Willebrand's disease there is an abnormality in a part of factor VIII known as von Willebrand factor (vWF). It is inherited in an autosomal dominant manner. It may be a quantitative or qualitative abnormality of vWF. In von Willebrand's disease there is an abnormality of platelet function and hence the bleeding time is prolonged. The PTTK may also be mildly increased.

Provan D, Chisholm M, Duncombe A, Singer C, Smith A
Oxford Handbook of Clinical Haematology Oxford University Press 1998

Mannucci PM, Tuddenham GD. The Haemophilias – From Royal Genes to Gene Therapy
NEJM 2001 344: 23; 1773–1779 & Editorial p1782

Question 20

A. false **B.** false **C.** true **D.** true **E.** false

Hypochromic microcytic red cell indices are seen classically in

iron deficiency anaemia
thalassaemia
sideroblastic anaemia

It can also be seen in chronic disease processes such as rheumatoid arthritis, however the anaemia associated with chronic disease is usually normochromic.

Investigation of unexplained hypochromic microcytic anaemia:

1. Blood film: red cell morphology, reticulocyte count
2. Iron studies: serum iron, TIBC, transferrin saturation, ferritin
3. Exclude bleeding in gastrointestinal or uterine tract

   Eg. endoscopy, colonoscopy, small bowel studies, 99mTc-labelled red cell scan, angiography
4. Marrow aspiration: stainable iron stores, ring sideroblasts
5. Urinary haemosiderin: increased in chronic haemolysis (eg Paroxysmal Nocturnal Haemoglobinuria)
6. Exclude malabsorption/malnutrition

Epstein RJ. Medicine for examinations
Churchill Livingstone

Question 21

A. true **B.** false **C.** false **D.** true **E.** true

Adverse prognostic features in Hodgkin's lymphoma

1. Subtype IV (lymphocyte depleted picture) at lymph node biopsy
2. Presence of B symptoms at presentation
3. Male
4. Older age

Clinical presentation of Hodgkin's disease:

1. B symptoms
   Stage A is Asymptomatic.
   Stage B: fever > 38°C
   sweats
   > 10% weight loss in the last 6 months

2 Pruritus (which is not a B symptom)

3. Pel-Ebstein (cyclical fever): classic but rare
4. Alcohol induced pain at sites of disease
5. Infection

Simplified Ann Arbor staging:

Stage 1: involvement of a single site (incl. extra nodal)

Stage 2: involvement of > 1 lymph node region on the same side of the diaphragm

Stage 3: Node involvement on both sides of the diaphragm

Stage 4: Extranodal disease (esp. marrow or liver).

Classical features on histologic subtypes of Hodgkin's disease:

1. Lymphocyte predominant: best prognosis, usually early stage (I, II) disease
2. Nodular sclerosing: indolent chemosensitive but relapsing disease, tends to affect young women, may cause bulky mediastinal adenopathy, spreads by contiguity, good prognosis unless bulky mediastinal disease
3. Mixed cellularity: often associated with occult splenic involvement, intermediate prognosis

4. Lymphocyte depletion: B symptoms (eg fever of unknown origin), adenopathy more widespread than other subtypes, may present with visceral involvement eg marrow fibrosis, osteoblastic bony disease (ivory vertebrae), spreads by dissemination to distant sites, worst prognosis.

Schwartz RS. Hodgkin's Disease, An Editorial
New England Journal of Medicine1997 337: 7; 453–458 & 459–465 and editorial 494–496

Tirelli U et al. Hodgkin's Disease: clinical presentation and treatment
Treatment Research 2001 104 247–265

Question 22

A. false **B.** false **C.** true **D.** false **E.** true

Peripheral polyneuropathy can occur during treatment with

Amphotericin
Chlorambucil
Cisplatin
Dapsone
Gold
Isoniazid
Metronidazole
Nitrofurantoin
Phenytoin
Vincristine

Burton JL, Healey CJ. Aids to Postgraduate Medicine
Sixth Edition, Churchill Livingstone 1994

Question 23

A. false **B.** true **C.** true **D.** true **E.** false

Non-steroidal anti-inflammatory drugs (NSAIDs) inhibit cyclo-oxygenase. This leads to a decrease in prostaglandin productions which are involved in the mediation of pain. There are 2 isoenzymes of cyclo-oxygenase, COX1 and COX2. COX2 is increased in the presence of inflammation and NSAIDs are thought to decrease inflammation through inhibition of this isoenzyme. COX 1 is located in the stomach and is responsible for the production of prostaglandins that protect the gastric mucosa. One of the major side effects of NSAIDs is gastric inflammation (gastritis) and bleeding hence the interest in the introduction of newer COX 2 specific NSAIDs. They have been used to some effect in controlling ACE inhibitor induced cough but the combination is associated with an increased risk of renal impairment. Cyclo-oxygenase 1 is expressed on platelets and so it is through this isoenzyme that impaired platelet aggregation is mediated.

Hawkey CJ et al. Review article: the gastrointestinal safety profile of rofecoxib, a highly selective inhibitor of cyclooxygenase-2 in humans. Aliment. Pharmacol. Ther. 2001 15: 1; 1–9

Question 24

A. true **B.** true **C.** false **D.** false **E.** true

Oramorph is a very effective analgesic. It is particularly useful at the initiation of therapy when modified release preparations are planned. By taking regular liquid morphine every 4 hours and using extra for breakthrough it is possible to calculate the dose of sustained release that will be required to control pain without giving too much and causing sedation. Diamorphine is more soluble than morphine and so can be given in a smaller volume hence it is used when subcutaneous administration is necessary. Morphine is excreted in urine. It therefore has an effective longer half-life in renal failure and so the interval of dosing should be increased. Opiates can induce coma in liver failure no matter what the cause of the liver failure is.

British National Formulary
BMA and Royal Pharmaceutical Society of Great Britain

Question 25

A. true **B.** true **C.** true **D.** true **E.** false

Photosensitivity occurs with many drugs. These include:

Amiodarone
Ciprofloxacin
Griseofulvin
Oral contraceptive
Phenothiazines
Retinoids
Sulphonamides
Sulphonylureas
Terbinafine – this antifungal agent has largely been replaced by griseofulvin

Tetracyclines
Thiazide diuretics

Burton JL, Healey CJ. Aids to Postgraduate Medicine
Sixth Edition, Churchill Livingstone 1994

Question 26

A. false **B.** false **C.** false **D.** true **E.** true

The appendices in the British National Formulary come well recommended whilst studying for this section of the exam. Nitrofurantoin is nephrotoxic and so should be avoided in even mild renal impairment. Mild renal impairment may be secondary to renal artery stenosis and so ACE inhibitors should be used with caution.

British National Formulary
BMA and Royal Pharmaceutical Society of Great Britain

Question 27

A. true **B.** false **C.** true **D.** true **E.** false

Aspirin overdose is the commonest type of salicylate poisoning. The clinical features

Respiratory alkalosis as a result of central respiratory stimulation
Nausea and vomiting
Tinnitus
Deafness
Sweating
Tachycardia
Later a metabolic acidosis occurs
Hypoglycaemia
Pulmonary oedema
Acute renal failure may occur

Treatment includes activated charcoal and correcting the electrolyte imbalance. A forced alkaline diuresis can be initiated but should be done in an ITU setting. Haemodialysis can be used in severe cases, usually at levels >750mg/litre.

Acute aspirin overdose: mechanisms of toxicity

Ther. Drug Monit. 1992 Dec 14(6): 441–451

Question 28

A. true **B.** false **C.** true **D.** false **E.** false

The correlation coefficient is between –1 and +1. A positive correlation means that as PEFR goes up; so does the height. The data is for heights from 160 and 190cm and the correlation coefficient applies only to this data. A correlation of zero IMPLIES no correlation.

PEFR is the first variable and so would go on the vertical axis

Driscoll P et al. Statistics 4: An introduction to estimation 1. Starting from Z J Accid Emerg Med 2000: 17; 409–415

Question 29

A. true **B.** false **C.** true **D.** false **E.** false

Juvenile chronic arthritis is also known as Still's disease. It is the commonest juvenile chronic arthritis accounting for 70% of cases. There is a bimodal distribution of age of onset – 2–5yrs and 10–15yrs. It is distinct from rheumatoid arthritis both clinically and immunologically ie. negative rheumatoid factor.

There are 3 subtypes

1. Systemic type
   usually <5 yrs
   high fever
   rash – patches of erythema on trunk or limbs which tends to occur in the evening or after a hot bath
   arthritis or arthralgia are often a minor feature at onset
   there may lymphadenopathy, splenomegaly or pericarditis
2. Pauciarticular
   Affects up to 4 large joints.
   They are prone to chronic iritis which can cause blindness without previous symptoms. This tends to be associated with positive ANA antibodies. If these are detected then the patient should have regular slit lamp examination.
3. Polyarticular

   This is a bilateral symmetrical polyarthropathy.

Diagnosis is made clinically. The symptoms and signs are:

high swinging fever
anaemia
raised ESR
high white cell count
joint swelling but little pain or tenderness

Eastmond CJ. Seronegative spondyloarthropathies
Oxford Textbook of Medicine. Oxford University Press

Question 30

A. false **B.** false **C.** true **D.** true **E.** false

Chondrocalcinosis is a cause of crystal arthropathy. The crystals are calcium pyrophosphate dihydrate. The condition causes an acute inflammatory arthritis which occurs in women as often as men. X-Ray may show linear calcification between and parallel to the articular surface. It is a recognized feature of:

Wilson's disease
Haemochromatosis
Idiopathic
hyper and hypoParathyroidism
Acromegaly
Diabetes mellitus
Ochronosis
Gout
(Mnemonic: WHIPADOG)

It is treated by rest, aspiration and steroid injections. NSAIDs are useful but are not as effective as in gout.

Schumacher HR Crystal induced arthritis: an overview
American Journal of Medicine 1996 100(2A): 46S–52S

Question 31

A. false **B.** true **C.** true **D.** false **E.** true

Vasculitis in rheumatoid arthritis is usually benign. It causes nailfold infarcts and mild sensory neuropathy usually in association with active joint disease. More rarely it can cause:

cutaneous ulceration
mononeuritis multiplex
mesenteric artery involvement which may cause ischaemic bowel

cerebral artery involvement causing strokes
coronary artery involvement causing myocardial ischaemia
The renal system is uninvolved.

Brooks PM Rheumatoid arthritis: aetiology and clinical features
Medicine 1998 26: 6; 28–31

Choy EHS et al. Cytokine pathways and joint inflammtion in Rheumatoid arthritis
NEJM 2001 344: 12; 907–916

Question 32

A. false **B.** true **C.** true **D.** true **E.** false

Guidelines for antibiotic prophylaxis for prevention of endocarditis.

Patients with heart valve lesions, septal defects, patent ductus or prosthetic valves require antibiotic prophylaxis when undergoing dental or upper respiratory tract procedures.

In addition patients with a prosthetic valve or previous history of endocarditis are deemed as high risk and also require prophylaxis when undergoing obstetric, gynaecological and gastro-intestinal procedures.

British National Formulary. British Medical Association and the Royal Pharmaceutical Society of Great Britain. London 2001

Question 33

A. true **B.** false **C.** true **D.** false **E.** true

For discussion of the various supraventricular tachycardias see Paper 3 Question 34.

Wolf Parkinson White (WPW) syndrome is important not only because of its clinical impact but also because of the opportunity to learn about electrical conduction in the heart. WPW is the 2nd commonest cause of paroxysmal SVT worldwide and curiously the commonest in China (>70% of cases). WPW affects roughly 1–3 people in every 1000. Affected individuals are born with an accessory pathway or bypass tract between the atria and ventricles that conducts more rapidly than the atrioventricular (AV) node leading to early ventricular depolarization. Evidence of this pre-excitation can be seen with a short pr interval and a slurred upstroke (the so-called delta wave) and widened QRS complex. Pre-excitation may be intermittent and patients may present with variable ECG patterns. Conduction through the pathway often occurs in a retrograde fashion, from ventricles to atria and thus the diagnosis may not be initially apparent with a normal ECG. Many patients suffer from symptomatic tachyarrhythmias the most common being paroxysmal supraventricular tachycardia due to a re-entrant circuit which begins with the impulse conducting from atria to ventricles via the AV node, then completes with conduction back to the atria by way of the accessory pathway. The onset of atrial fibrillation or flutter may precipitate ventricular tachycardia or fibrillation. Patients may present for the first time with palpitations, pre syncope, syncope or sudden death. For diagnostic and therapeutic work cardiologists can perform electrophysiologic studies (catheter based mapping) and radio-frequency ablation of the accessory pathway as definitive treatment.

Occasionally patients with WPW have concomitant congenital heart disease; 10% of patients with Ebstein's anomaly have WPW syndrome. Other associated heart disease includes:

Atrial septal defect

Ventricular septal defect

Coronary sinus diverticulae

Corrected transposition of the great vessels

3–4% of first-degree relatives have evidence of pre-excitation. There is a familial form of WPW syndrome that is autosomal dominant. Mitochondrial inheritance is rare. The syndrome may also be inherited with other Mendelian cardiac and non-cardiac disorders such as familial atrial septal defects, familial hypokalaemic periodic paralysis and tuberose sclerosis and autosomal dominant familial hypertrophic cardiomyopathy. Recent studies focussing on families with familial WPW syndrome confirmed an autosomal dominant pattern with complete penetrance and incomplete (variable) expression. A causative mutation was identified in a protein kinase gene (PRKAG2) on chromosome 7.

Gollob MH et al. Identification of a Gene Responsible for Familial Wolff-Parkinson-White Syndrome. NEJM 2001 344: 24; 1823–1831

Question 34

A. false **B.** false **C.** false **D.** false **E.** false

Rheumatic fever is the major cause of mitral stenosis and as such the incidence is now declining. Other causes include connective tissue disorders, Hurlers syndrome, prosthetic valve, and carcinoid. Stenosis may be due to the valve leaflets thickening and calcifying, the chordae shortening and fusing, or the commissures fusing.

Dyspnoea occurs as the left atrial pressure rises and is transmitted to the pulmonary circulation causing a raised wedge pressure and secondary pulmonary hypertension. Acute pulmonary oedema may develop. Other symptoms include fatigue, haemoptysis, systemic embolization (20–30%), chronic bronchitis, chest pain, palpitations, right heart failure, hoarsness, dysphagia or left lung collapse due to left atrial enlargement. Physical signs include malar flush, loud S1, opening snap due to mobile leaflets, rumbling diastolic murmur, tapping apex (not displaced) and secondary pulmonary hypertension and tricuspid regurgitation. Pregnacy, new atrial fibrillation, exercise, pneumonia, and anaesthesia can all cause an acute deterioration in symptoms. Echocardiography is useful in mitral stenosis as the mobility of the mitral leaflets is easily assessed and the severity of the stenosis can be estimated. It can also distinguish mitral stenosis from left atrial myxoma, HOCM, ASD with flow murmur, and aortic regurgitation which can all cause a similar clinical picture.

Treatment is conservative until patients develop NYHA class III or IV symptoms at which stage surgical intervention should be considered. The options are valvuloplasty, valvotomy, or valve replacement.

Swanton RH. Cardiology 4th Ed. Blackwell Scientific Publications Ltd. Oxford

Question 35

A. false **B.** false **C.** false **D.** true **E.** true

The ductus arteriosus connects the pulmonary artery to the aorta in utero. It usually closes within the first month after birth though can remain persistently open, with the development of a left-to-right shunt. If significant this can cause LV hypertrophy, pulmonary hypertension, symptoms of LVF, and eventually Eisenmenger's syndrome due to shunt reversal.

Physical signs include differential cyanosis (feet>hands), collapsing pulse, continuous machinery murmur left 2nd I.S., left venticular hypertrophy, mitral diastolic flow murmur.

Ledingham J (Ed). Concise Oxford textbook of Medicine. 2000 Oxford University Press, Oxford

Question 36

A. false **B.** false **C.** true **D.** false **E.** false

See Paper 2: Question 35

Question 37

A. false **B.** true **C.** true **D.** false **E.** false

Ocular abnormalities are not characteristic of Alzheimer's disease, Duchenne muscular dystrophy and Motor neurone disease.

Wernicke's encephalopathy represents the triad of cerebellar ataxia, ophthalmoplegia (most commonly nystagmus or VI nerve palsy), and confusion. It is due to thiamine deficiency which causes degeneration of the mamillary bodies and associated subthalamic structures. It usually occurs in combination with Korsakoff's syndrome of severe amnesia with confabulation and lack of insight, though one clinical picture may predominate. The diagnosis is predominantly based on the clinical findings but is supported by the finding of reduced red cell transketolase activity. Treatment is with thiamine replacement which should be started prior to giving a carbohydrate load as this can precipitate a deterioration. Wernicke's disease usually improves following thiamine replacement whilst the outlook for established Korsakoff's syndrome is poor.

Causes of Wernicke's encephalopathy include

Alcoholism
Gastric cancer
Gastric surgery
Hyperemesis gravidarum
Haemodialysis
Pyruvate dehydrogenase deficiency

Zabaran C et al. Wenicke-Korsakoff Syndrome. Postgraduate Medical Journal 1997 73(855): 27–31

Question 38

A. false **B.** false **C.** false **D.** true **E.** false

Guillain-Barré syndrome is the commonest clinical presentation of the autoimmune inflammatory neuropathies. Other variants include the Miller-Fisher syndrome and chronic relapsing neuropathy. Guillain-Barré syndrome has an annual incidence of 1:50,000, and in 2/3rds of cases is preceded by a respiratory or gastrointestinal infection, such as Campylobacter jejuni, Mycoplasma pneumoniae, CMV or EBV. The typical presentation is with weakness of the upper and lower limbs which may progress for up to 4 weeks and is often accompanied by neuropathic back pain. Reflexes are usually absent, sensory loss may occur, and autonomic, respiratory muscle, and cranial nerves are often involved.

The diagnosis is made on the basis of a typical clinical picture, a typically elevated CSF protein, and demyelination on nerve conduction studies. However early in the disease reflexes may be present and the CSF protein normal as the myelin sheaths have not broken down. In a small proportion of cases axonal degeneration occurs which indicates a poorer outcome. Antibodies to the membrane-bound glycolipid, ganglioside GM1, is found in Guillain-Barré syndrome but is not sufficiently sensitive or specific to be used routinely. Treatment is mainly supportive with attention being paid to the complications of respiratory failure, thromboembolic disease, and cardiac arrhythmias. Both plasmapheresis and IV immunoglobulin are equally effective in reducing the length of paralysis and improving outcome and one should be started as soon as possible after the diagnosis is made. Combination therapy is no more effective than monotherapy with either modality. In general 75% make a good to full recovery, 15% remain severely disabled at one year, and 10% die.

Miller-Fisher syndrome is the uncommon combination of ophthalmoplegia, ataxia, and absent reflexes in the absence of peripheral weakness. Antibodies to ganglioside GQ1b are a sensitive and specific marker for the disorder. Treatment is as for Guillain-Barre syndrome.

Causes of acute peripheral neuropathy include

Guillain-Barré
Vasculitis
Porphyria
Sarcoid
Alcohol
Lead
Isoniazid

Taxol
Vincristine
Organophosphates
Arsenic
Diphtheria
HIV
Lyme disease
Polio

Hadden RDM, et al. Autoimmune inflammatory neuropathy
J R Coll Physicians Lond 1999 33: 219–224

Question 39

A. false **B.** false **C.** true **D.** false **E.** true

Alzheimers disease is characterized by a gradual decline in functional and cognitive ability associated with progressive memory loss. The prevalence increases with age from 3% at the age of 65 to 47% at the age of 85. Ageing is the primary risk factor though there is also an association with female sex, head injury, Down's syndrome, and family history. A small number of cases arising before the age of 60 are inherited in an autosomal dominant manner due to mutations in the gene for amyloid precursor protein or the genes for presenilin 1 or 2. There is also an association with allele 4 of the Apo E lipoprotein gene which may be inherited or occur sporadically. This may be the basis for the early onset of disease seen in patients suffering from Down's syndrome.

Clinically there is a gradual decline in cognitive function associated with increasing difficulty in performing routine daily functions such as cooking a meal. Behavioural changes are common as is co-existing depression. In end-stage disease patients may be mute and death usually results from co-morbid conditions such as pneumonia or pulmonary embolism. The average life-expectancy is 8–10 years following the onset of dementia. The diagnosis relies on typical clinical features and the exclusion of other disorders such as hypothyroidism and cerebrovascular disease.

The neuro-pathological basis appears to be neuronal cell death associated with a reduction in acetylcholine levels. Post-mortem examinations reveal senile plaques, comprised of extracellular deposits of beta-amyloid protein and degenerating neuronal components, and intracellular neurofibrillary tangles, composed of abnormally phosphorylated tau protein. These are distributed throughout the cerebral cortex in markedly increased numbers compared to non-demented age-matched controls.

Treatment has focused on augmenting cholinergic transmission. Donepezil is a selective reversible inhibitor of acetylcholinesterase, that has been licensed for use in mild to moderate dementia. It has a small but significant benefit in delaying the progression of the disease. HRT and NSAIDs may have a protective effect against the development of Alzheimers.

Carr DB, et al. Current concepts in the pathogenesis of Alzheimers disease American Journal of Medicine 1997 103(3A) Supplement 22: 3S–10S

Question 40

A. false **B.** true **C.** true **D.** true **E.** true

Factors associated with an increased risk of suicide:

Evidence of intent
- Planning
- Precautions to avoid discovery
- No attempt to obtain help
- Violent method eg. hanging
- Final act eg. note
  - Continuing wish to die
  - Previous history of self-harm

Psychiatric disorder

Alcoholism

Social and environmental
- Recent bereavement
- Social isolation
- Unemployed
- Older age
- Male sex; women are more likely to attempt suicide, but men are more likely to intend to kill themselves

Criminal record

Suicide and deliberate self-harm. In Gelder M, Mayou R, Geddes J, eds. Psychiatry, Oxford: Oxford University Press, 1999.

Question 41

A. true **B.** true **C.** false **D.** false **E.** false

The following are features of an acute episode of schizophrenia (positive symptoms)

Appearance and behaviour
Restless, noisy and inconsistent
Preoccupied and withdrawn

Mood
Mood changes
Emotionally blunted

Thought disorders
See Paper 1 Question 43

Hallucinations
Usually auditory, often persecutory. (Visual hallucinations would be more suggestive of acute confusional state/delirium)

Delusions
Primary and secondary

Impaired attention

Lack of insight

Patients tend to be orientated in time and have a complete memory of recent events.

Primary delusions occur spontaneously, with conviction and with no obvious related event. These are rare but are highly suggestive of schizophrenia. Secondary delusions arise almost understandably from another event, such as a hallucination, a mood or another delusion.

Schizophrenia and related disorders. In Gelder M, Mayou R, Geddes J, eds. Psychiatry, Oxford: Oxford University Press, 1999.

Question 42

A. false **B.** true **C.** false **D.** false **E.** true

Depression and dementia are often found in the elderly, and there are many common features.

Symptoms of depression in the elderly that distinguish it from dementia:

Poor memory and concentration; patients may complain excessively about memory loss

Denial of depressive symptoms

Biological depressive symptoms occur

Disturbed sleep,
Loss of motivation and appetite
Pessimistic outlook
Erectile impotence
Morning worsening of mood (in dementia there is evening worsening of confusion)

Acute or subacute onset, over weeks or months

Impaired attention

Impaired or inconsistent cognitive tests

'Dont knows' rather than near miss responses to questions are common.

Faecal incontinence and other disinhibited behaviour are suggestive of dementia. Often the two (dementia and depression) are impossible to distinguish, and in fact may co-exist. Depression in the elderly with symptoms similar to or suggestive of dementia is often described as pseudodementia or depressive pseudodementia.

Hodges JR. Dementia; an introduction. In Weatherall DJ, Ledingham JGG, Warrell DA, eds. Oxford Textbook of Medicine, Oxford: Oxford University Press, 1996.

Question 43

A. false **B.** false **C.** false **D.** false **E.** false

Definition of Anorexia nervosa – three features are required:

1. Active maintenance of a low body weight (around 15% below estimated normal for height, age and sex). Achieving weight loss is by dieting, fasting, excessive exercise or self induced vomiting. Patients with IDDM may underuse or omit insulin.

2. Characteristic attitudes to shape and weight such as "relentless pursuit of thinness" or "morbid fear of fatness" are present. This feature is often more striking than the first but occurs some time after the initial weight loss.

3. The third diagnostic feature is amenorrhoea (in postmenarchal females who are not taking an oral contraceptive).

Anorexia nervosa usually occurs in women aged 10–30 in Western cultures where thinness is considered attractive and its incidence is 0.24–14.6 per 100,000 females. Less than 10% are males and it is also uncommon amongst non-Caucasians. Adolescents comprise the highest risk group. More patients present from higher socio-economic groups. Contrary to the state suggested by the diagnostic label patients do not lose their appetite except in very long standing cases. Psychological manifestations include depressed mood, lability of mood, irritability, and anxiety and obsessional symptoms related to eating. In more chronic cases there may be hopelessness and thoughts of suicide. There is preoccupation with thoughts about food, eating, shape, and weight, and concentration may be impaired. As weight falls outside interests tend to decline and social withdrawal may be marked. Often patients have no symptoms at all but if they are questioned closely they may have the following:

1. heightened sensitivity to cold
2. a variety of gastrointestinal symptoms such as constipation, fullness after eating, bloatedness, and vague abdominal pains
3. restlessness, lack of energy, low sexual appetite, and early morning wakening
4. in females who are not taking an oral contraceptive, amenorrhoea is by definition present
5. infertility.

Examination:

1. the degree of emaciation may be striking. Weakness (hypokalaemia) and myopathy (nutritional) may also be present
2. growth may be stunted in those with a prepubertal onset and there may be a failure of breast development
3. unlike patients with hypopituitarism, axillary and pubic hair is preserved and there is no breast atrophy
4. a fine downy lanugo hair may be present on the back, arms, and side of face. The skin is usually dry and the hands and feet are cold
5. blood pressure and pulse are low, hypothermia may be present
6. there may be dependent oedema

An ECG may show arrhythmias or a prolonged QT interval

Increased in anorexia nervosa: cortisol (diurnal variation is lost), growth hormone, cholesterol, serum beta carotene

Unchanged: amino acids, vitamin levels, prolactin, androgens

Reduced: LH and FSH, and LHRH, potassium, ESR, somatomedin C, blood glucose, TSH (low or normal), T4 and T3. A normocytic normochromic anaemia is found in a minority of patients and is sometimes attributable to a low intake of iron or folate. Note that a life threatening hypoglycaemia can rarely occur and this may not present itself in the usual fashion if there is an impaired sympathetic response. The answer in stem c is false as this is not characteristic in anorexics.

Complications other than amenorrhoea in anorexia nervosa

1. dental caries
2. gastric dilatation or atrophy
3. constipation
4. renal calculi
5. osteoporosis

Stoving RK. Hangaard J. Hansen-Nord M. Hagen C. A review of endocrine changes in anorexia nervosa. Journal of Psychiatric Research 1999 33(2): 139–152

Question 44

A. false **B.** true **C.** false **D.** true **E.** true

The fact that atenolol can cause bronchospasm should not be in doubt. It is not entirely cardiospecific and should be used with care if at all in patients prone to bronchospasm.

NSAIDs can exacerbate asthma in a small percentage of patients. This is a type I hypersensitivity reaction; rashes, angioedema and other allergic phenomena may occur.

The phenomenon of paradoxical bronchospasm after inhalation aerosols is well described, although the cause is as yet unknown as this occurs quite rarely. Long-acting bronchodilators like salmeterol seem to be more likely to cause this problem.

Risk factors for unexpected death in asthma:

Recent discharge from hospital
Overdependency on inhaled beta-agonists
Non-compliance or under utilization of inhaled or systemic steroids
Intravenous administration of aminophylline in patients already receiving maintenance oral theophylline.

Lung infiltrates; upper or lower zone on CXR

Upper zone:
- Silicosis
- Coal workers pneumoconiosis
- Histocytosis X
- Aspergillosis
- Ankylosing Spondylitis
- Tuberculosis

Lower Zone:
- Bronchiectasis
- Rheumatoid arthritis
- Asbestosis
- Scleroderma
- Haemosiderosis
- Idiopathic pulmonary fibrosis
- Others; radiation, cytotoxic drugs

Cocchetto DM. Sykes RS. Spector S. Paradoxical bronchospasm after use of inhalation aerosols: a review of the literature. Journal of Asthma 1991. 28(1): 49–53

British National Formulary. London: British Medical Association and the Royal Pharmaceutical Society of Great Britain 2001

Question 45

A. true **B.** false **C.** true **D.** true **E.** true

This question has been answered in Paper 3 Question 44. Myringitis is inflammation of the eardrum. Mycoplasma causes erythema multiforme; erythema marginatum is a major criterion for the diagnosis of Rheumatic fever.

Other causes of Erythema multiforme:

- Herpes simplex
- Drugs: Sulphonamides, Sulphonylureas, barbiturates
- Other infection: Streptococcus, Yersiniosis, tuberculosis
- Connective tissue diseases: SLE
- Neoplasia (uncommon)
- Usually no cause is found.

Epstein RJ. Medicine for examinations. 3rd Ed. Churchill Livingstone, London, 1996.

Question 46

A. false **B.** true **C.** true **D.** true **E.** false

Indications for bronchoalveolar lavage:

Diagnostic lavage
Opportunistic infections, eg Pneumocystis
Alveolar haemorrhagic syndromes
Alveolar proteinosis
Dust disease, eg Asbestosis

Prognostic lavage
Fibrosing alveolitis (Increased neutrophils in active disease, worse prognosis if >10% neutrophils, better prognosis if >25% lymphocytosis)
Sarcoid (Excess of helper-T cells worse prognosis)
Hypersensitivity pneumonitis
ARDS
Drug induced lung disease

Therapeutic lavage
Pulmonary alveolar proteinosis
Cystic fibrosis/bronchiectasis
Asthma with mucous plugging

Epstein RJ. Medicine for examinations. 3rd Ed. Churchill Livingstone, London, 1996.

Question 47

A. false **B.** false **C.** false **D.** false **E.** true

Pneumoconiosis is the generic term for any inhaled dust that becomes lodged in the lungs irrespective of the effects. Chest x-ray evidence is needed to diagnose this.

Silo-fillers disease is a toxic pneumonitis caused by the nitrogen dioxide released by grain products held in silos.

Isocyanates are the most common cause of occupational asthma, as a result of paint spraying of coaches etc. Inhalation of irritant gases such as chlorine results in pulmonary oedema.

Most cases of mesothelioma develop 20–40 years after exposure to even small amounts of blue (crocidolite) or brown (amosite) asbestos.

Cases of work related respiratory disease in order of frequency:

Occupational asthma:
Isocyanates
Laboratory animals
Grain from baking and milling

Non-malignant pleural disease:
Asbestos
Mesothelioma

Pneumoconiosis:
Silicosis
Coal-workers pneumoconiosis

Inhalation accidents:
Chlorine
Lung cancer
Infectious disease
Extrinsic allergic alveolitis (See Paper 2 Question 47)
Bronchitis
Building-related illness
Byssinosis

Ira Madan. ABC of Work Related Disorders: Occupational Asthma and other Respiratory Diseases. BMJ 1996 313: 291–294.

Ross DJ, Sallie BA, McDonald JC. SWORD'94: surveillance of work-related and occupational respiratory disease in the UK. Occup Med 1995 45: 175–178.

Beckett WS. Occupational Respiratory Diseases
NEJM 2000 342 6: 406–413

Question 48

A. true **B.** false **C.** true **D.** true **E.** true

The features of coeliac disease have been discussed on Paper 1 Question 48 and Paper 3 Question 49. Dermatitis herpetiformis is associated with coeliac disease although often presents as a separate entity with a gluten sensitive rash in the absence of an enteropathy. It is an indication for a small bowel biopsy.

Causes of splenic atrophy: sickle cell disease, coeliac disease, dermatitis herpetiformis, ulcerative colitis, Crohn's disease, essential thrombocytopenia, Fanconis anaemia and old age. The mechanism of splenic atrophy is unknown.

Classification of oral ulcers:

Recurrent oral ulcers
Minor, major aphthous, and herpetiform, Behcet's syndrome

Microbial infection
Primary and recurrent herpes simplex infection, Herpes zoster infection, acute ulcerative gingivostomatitis, Tuberculosis, Syphilis

Neoplastic ulcers
Carcinoma, Leukaemia

Haematological disorders
Anaemia, Neutropenia, agranulocytosis

Dermatological disorders
Erosive lichen planus, Pemphigus, Benign mucous membrane pemphigoid, Erythema multiforme and Stevens-Johnson syndrome

Reiter's syndrome

Granulomatous disorders
Histiocytosis X, Wegener's granulomatosis

Iatrogenic agents
Drug allergy, Drug-induced agranulocytosis, Cytotoxic drugs, Radiotherapy

Trauma
Denture, teeth, or foreign body, Chemical

Feighery C. Clinical Review: Coeliac disease.
BMJ 1999 319: 236–239.

Question 49

A. false **B.** true **C.** true **D.** true **E.** false

Stress was previously thought to be a major factor in the aetiology of duodenal ulcer (DU) but is now thought to be much less important. The discovery of Helicobacter pylori has revolutionised the understanding of peptic ulcer pathogenesis and therapy. Most patients with a DU will have a specific cause, probably either H pylori or non-steroidal anti-inflammatory drugs (NSAIDs) so even if treated with H2 receptor antagonists it is likely that if these are discontinued and the underlying cause is unchanged that the ulcer will return. This has been confirmed in a systematic overview, the median 12 month DU recurrence rate was 67% if H pylori persisted, and 6% if eradicated. The reduction in gastric acid secretion after eradication of H pylori forms part of the evidence that H pylori is instrumental in the pathogenesis of DU though it is likely that other factors also play a part. The CLO test, histological biopsy and serology are other methods of identifying H pylori infection. Any would be adequate in the appropriate setting (eg inflammation such as duodenitis, erosions or frank ulceration) to prompt eradication. As H pylori infection is so likely in a non-NSAID DU, some authorities would counsel eradication whether or not infection is proven, although this is not current accepted practise.

Chiba N, Hunt RH. Ulcer disease and Helicobacter pylori infection: aetiology and treatment. McDonald J, Feagan B, Burroughs A, eds. Evidence Based Gastroenterology and Hepatology, London: BMJ Books, 1999.

Question 50

A. true **B.** false **C.** false **D.** true **E.** false

There is a relative risk of up to 6 for Crohn's disease in smokers in contrast to ulcerative colitis where smoking is protective. Crohn's is less likely to occur after surgery where patients stop smoking. Crohn's disease is more common in developed, Western countries, and is rare in India, Africa and South America, although there is difficulty in diagnosing Crohn's disease in areas where intestinal tuberculosis is common. Coeliac disease would be the most likely cause of malabsorption syndrome in a 15-year old. Coeliac disease probably has a prevalence of about 1 in 300 in this country, whereas Crohn's disease prevalence is around 1:1,500. Aminosalicylic acid therapy for Crohn's is generally only suitable in colonic disease, although theoretically terminal ileal disease may respond to some preparations. HLA associations of Crohn's disease are generally weak, with the following suggested: HLA DR1, DQw5 and, in patients with associated ankylosing spondylitis, HLA B27. Monozygotic twins have a concordance rate of up to 70%.

Yamamoto T. Keighley MR. Smoking and disease recurrence after operation for Crohn's disease. British Journal of Surgery 2000 Apr. 87(4): 398–404

Thomas GA. Rhodes J. Green JT. Richardson C. Role of smoking in inflammatory bowel disease: implications for therapy. Postgraduate Medical Journal 2000 May. 76(895): 273–279

Question 51

A. false **B.** false **C.** true **D.** true **E.** false

Most patients with carcinoma of the stomach have advanced disease at the time of presentation so, in addition to pain, they have anorexia and weight loss. 50% have nausea and vomiting which can be severe if the tumour is near the pylorus, whereas dysphagia can occur with tumours involving the fundus.

Gross haematemesis is unusual but anaemia from occult blood loss is frequent. Patients can also present with problems related to metastases, in particular abdominal swelling due to ascites or jaundice due to liver involvement. Metastases, however, can occur to bone, brain, and lungs, producing appropriate symptoms. A palpable lymph node is sometimes found in the left supraclavicular fossa (Virchow sign). Signs of metastases are present in up to a third of patients.

Carcinoma of the stomach is the cancer most frequently associated with dermatomyositis and acanthosis nigricans. Endoscopy is the investigation of choice.

There is an increased risk of gastric cancer in:

1. native residents of Japan, Chile, Costa Rica (risk continues when migration occurs to a low-risk area, although decreases with successive generations)
2. coal miners and some chemical workers (no specific hazards have been identified)
3. lower socio-economic groups
4. common variable immune deficiency (50-fold)
5. blood group A
6. gastritis associated with H pylori
7. a diet deficient in fruit and green and yellow vegetables
8. poor diet with large amounts of salt
9. cigarette smoking
10. nitrosamines via high dietary or water nitrate.
11. reduced (absent) gastric acidity; pernicious anaemia and partial gastrectomy.

Vitamin C reduces the risk of gastric cancer. Although there is more to be learnt about the natural history of gastric cancer, it seems that it must take at least 15 years post-gastrectomy for the tumour to develop.

Eurogast Study Group (1993). An international association between H pylori infection and gastric cancer. Lancet 1993 341: 1359–1362

Craven JL (1991). Gastric cancer. Current opinion in gastroenterology 7, 933–8

Question 52

A. false **B.** false **C.** false **D.** false **E.** true

Causes of polyuria-polydipsia syndromes

Cranial diabetes insipidus:

Familial
dominant inheritance (occasionally autosomal recessive)
DIDMOAD (diabetes mellitus, diabetes insipidus, optic atrophy and deafness or Wolfram syndrome autosomal recessive)

Acquired
idiopathic
trauma (neurosurgery, head injury)
neoplasia (craniopharyngiomas, hypothalamic metastasis, large pituitary tumour)
infection (meningitis, encephalitis)
vascular (sickle-cell, Sheehans syndrome)
granuloma (sarcoid)

Nephrogenic diabetes insipidus:

Familial (X linked recessive)

Acquired
idiopathic
metabolic (hypercalcaemia, hypokalaemia)
vascular (sickle cell)
osmotic diuresis (glycosuria, post-obstructive uropathy)
drugs (lithium, demeclocycline, amphotericin)

The clinical manifestations of cranial diabetes insipidus (DI) are polyuria, nocturia, excessive thirst and drinking water. Children often present with enuresis. Most patients have a partial deficiency of vasopressin. Patients with cranial diabetes insipidus usually maintain serum sodium and plasma osmolality within the normal ranges as they have an intact thirst mechanism, and are able to drink water freely.

Cranial DI may be masked by glucocorticoid hormone deficiency due to either hypopituitarism or primary adrenal failure. Cortisol is essential for the maximum diluting function of the distal nephron.

Symptoms occur often during pregnancy due to increased clearance of arginine vasopressin caused by vasopressinase, a circulating enzyme that is of placental origin.

Nephrogenic DI is usually partial with mild symptoms. Again serum sodium and plasma osmolality are usually within the normal range, although urine osmolality is low. Nephrogenic DI is where the renal tubules are either completely or partially resistant to the action of Vasopressin.

Primary polydipsia (PPD) patients drink large quantities or fluid in excess of body requirements, usually due to psychological disturbance. Nocturia is less of a feature than DI, as renal function is normal, and they do not drink through the night. Patients with this drink faster than they can get rid of water, despite suppression of vasopressin, and their serum sodium tends to be lower than that in cranial and nephrogenic DI, although it often still tends to be within the reference range. Patients with PPD can drink up to 20 litres per 24hr and still have a normal sodium

Bayliss PH. Water and sodium homeostasis and their disorders. In Weatherall DJ, Ledingham JGG, Warrell DA, eds. Oxford Textbook of Medicine, Oxford: Oxford University Press, 1996.

Question 53

A. true **B.** true **C.** false **D.** true **E.** true

This question has partly been answered in Paper 5 Question 54. Hemiplegia, and short stroke-like episodes are separate from diabetic neuropathy, and are neuroglycopenic symptoms as are headaches. Night sweats and mood changes, particularly aggression, are typical of adrenergic symptoms. Foot drop is not caused by hypoglycaemia as the neuroglycopenic symptoms tend to give central symptoms and signs, rather than the diabetic mononeuropathy causing foot-drop or peripheral polyneuropathy.

Bell JI, Hockaday TDR. Diabetes Mellitus. In Weatherall DJ, Ledingham JGG, Warrell DA, eds. Oxford Textbook of Medicine, Oxford: Oxford University Press, 1996.

Question 54

A. true **B.** false **C.** true **D.** false **E.** true

Prolactin is synthesized by the human anterior pituitary gland from the fifth week of gestation. Its secretion varies under different physiological conditions and is regulated by hypothalamic dopamine, which inhibits its release in a tonic fashion and by prolactin-releasing factors. Concentrations are higher in normal premenopausal women than men, and rise during menarche in girls, and during pregnancy in both mother and foetus. Prolactin rises with suckling, greatest response being after delivery. Hyperprolactinaemia occurs with disruption of the hypothalamus, the hypothalamus stalk, or administration of drugs that interfere with dopamine synthesis or action. In patients with hypothyroidism there may be mild hyperprolactinaemia, due to increased hypothalamic TRH secretion.

Physiology of prolactin:

Although it acts at various sites the main site of action is in the mammary gland where it stimulates lactation, and has a large role in breast development during pregnancy in addition to other hormones such as oestrogen and progesterone as well as to some extent insulin, cortisol and thyroxine. Lactation is inhibited until the high concentrations seen with pregnancy of oestrogen and progesterone fall at parturition and the action of prolactin becomes unopposed. Dopamine agonists can be used to inhibit prolactin secretion, and thereby lactation, after delivery. The physiological functions of prolactin at other sites are poorly characterized, but it is known to regulate dopamine turnover and affect gonadotrophin secretion in the hypothalamus; both the hyperprolactinaemia of pregnancy and lactation, and pathological hyperprolactinaemia are associated with suppression of the hypothalamic-pituitary-gonadal axis. This is likely to be due to prolactin-mediated inhibition of pulsatile gonadotrophin releasing hormone (GnRH) secretion, resulting in disorganized gonadotrophin secretion and dysregulation of gonadal function.

Thorner MO. Anterior pituitary disorders. In Weatherall DJ, Ledingham JGG, Warrell DA, eds. Oxford Textbook of Medicine, Oxford: Oxford University Press, 1996.

Question 55

A. true **B.** true **C.** false **D.** true **E.** true

Classification of osteoporosis:

Common forms, unassociated with other disease
Idiopathic osteoporosis (juvenile and adult)
Type I osteoporosis
Type II osteoporosis

Osteoporosis as a common feature
Hypogonadism
Cushing's syndrome; spontaneous and iatrogenic
Hyperparathyroidism
Thyrotoxicosis
Malabsorption
Scurvy
Calcium deficiency
Immobilization
Chronic heparin administration
Systemic mastocytosis
Adult hypophosphatasia
Associated with other metabolic bone diseases

Osteoporosis as a feature of heritable disorders of connective tissue
Osteogenesis imperfecta
Homocystinuria due to cystathionine synthase deficiency
Ehlers-Danlos syndrome
Marfan's syndrome

Osteoporosis is associated but pathogenesis is not understood
Rheumatoid arthritis
Cigarette smoking
Malnutrition
Alcoholism
Epilepsy
Primary Biliary cirrhosis
Diabetes mellitus
Chronic obstructive pulmonary disease
Menkes syndrome

In thyrotoxicosis bone turnover is excessive, bone resorption being increased to a greater extent than bone formation, and after many years of thyroid overactivity significant osteoporosis may occur. As thyrotoxicosis is often recognized early, significant bone disease is uncommon. It may be seen in thyroxine addicts. There is some evidence that alcohol has a direct effect on osteoblasts, although there are plenty of reasons why alcohol addicts should have osteoporosis. Cigarette smoking and being thin are also said to cause osteoporosis.

Thiazides reduce calcium excretion and femoral neck fracture rate and have been used in the treatment of osteoporosis.

Kanis JA. Disorders of Calcium Metabolism. In Weatherall DJ, Ledingham JGG, Warrell DA, eds. Oxford Textbook of Medicine, Oxford: Oxford University Press, 1996.

Question 56

A. true **B.** true **C.** true **D.** false **E.** true

Psoriasis causes

pitting
hyperkeratosis
loss of the nail
onycholysis

Other causes of abnormalities of the nail or nail bed include

fungal infections
bacterial infections
lichen planus
alopecia areata
dermatitis
iron deficiency, haemochromatosis and hyperthyroidism cause koilonychia
yellow nail syndrome

Hypoalbuminaemia causes paired narrow white transverse bands known as Muehrcke's lines.

Hypoparathyroidism is associated with hypocalcaemia which is a cause of Beau's lines

Splinter haemorrhages are usually the result of trauma but can occur in infective endocarditis

de Berker D Nails
Medicine 2000 25: 8; 26–29

Question 57

A. true **B.** true **C.** false **D.** true **E.** true

Post-streptococcal glomerulonephritis usually presents 2 weeks after a streptococcal infection with acute onset nephritic or nephrotic syndrome. It has a peak incidence in children between 2 and 10 years though can present at any age. Only certain nephritogenic strains of streptococci are associated with glomerulonephritis of which pharyngeal infection with type 12 streptococcus is the most common. The pathogenic mechanism is largely unknown but probably involves an inflammatory response to renal deposition of streptococcal antigens (possibly streptokinase) with subsequent immune-complex formation and deposition of C3 and IgG. On microscopy there is a diffuse proliferation of mesangial and endothelial cells with crescent formation in severe cases. Subendothelial and subepithelial deposits can be seen on electron microscopy.

It is an acute and reversible disease that results in spontaneous recovery in most patients. The long-term prognosis is generally good though in some series up to 20% of subjects have developed chronic renal impairment.

Hricik DE et al. Glomerulonephritis
NEJM 1998 339(13): 888–899

Question 58

A. true **B.** true **C.** true **D.** true **E.** false

Polyuria occurs in all of the above except for subjects receiving NSAIDS.

In the acute setting NSAIDs inhibit renal vasodilatory prostaglandins, reducing renal blood flow, and thus water excretion. This can lead to renal failure which is largely reversible on stopping the drug. Risk factors for the development of acute renal failure on NSAIDs include old age, diabetes, renal impairment, and hypertension. Rarely NSAIDs can lead to the development of interstitial nephritis. Chronic usage may be associated with the development of renal papillary necrosis and subsequent chronic renal failure, typical of analgesic nephropathy. However classical analgesic nephropathy is more strongly associated with long-term usage of a combination of phenacetin, paracetamol, or aspirin with codeine or caffeine.

De Broe ME et al. Analgesic nephropathy
NEJM 1998 338(7): 446–452

Question 59

A. false **B.** false **C.** true **D.** false **E.** true

See Paper 1 Question 56

Question 60

A. false **B.** false **C.** false **D.** true **E.** false

Membranous nephropathy usually presents with heavy proteinuria, accounting for approximately 25% of adult cases of the nephrotic syndrome. Microscopic haematuria does occur in up to 20% of cases though macroscopic haematuria is rare in adults. There is a 3:1 male to female ratio with the majority of patients presenting between the age of 30 and 50 years. It is most commonly idiopathic though 25% of cases are secondary to drugs, carcinoma, lymphoma, SLE or chronic infection with hepatitis B or C. 10% of patients on long-term gold or penicillamine develop membranous nephropathy which may persist for up to two years following cessation of treatment. On light microscopy there is diffuse thickening of the glomerular basement membrane with subepithelial spikes. This is due to subepithelial deposits of IgG and C3. In general the course of the disease is fairly benign with recent studies showing 90% of patients with all cause membranous nephropathy to have functioning kidneys after 5 years of follow up. However patients who present with severe nephrotic syndrome, poor renal function, or tubulointerstitial fibrosis on biopsy may follow a worse course with a more rapid deterioration in renal function. Treatment is with steroids +/– chlorambucil or cyclophosphamide though the risks of immunosuppressive therapy must be weighed against the relatively good prognosis the disease carries. Thus treatment should be reserved for patients in the subgroup described above with a worse prognosis or with deteriorating renal function. Renal vein thrombosis is common in association with membranous glomerulonephritis and must be considered in any patient with a sudden deterioration in renal function.

Zucchelli P, Pasquali S. Membranous Nephropathy.
Davidson AM et al. Oxford Textbook of Clinical Nephrology. 2nd Ed. 1998.

Paper 5 Answers

Question 1

A. false **B.** true **C.** false **D.** true **E.** true

See Paper 4 Question 2 for a discussion on Marfan's syndrome.

Question 2

A. false **B.** true **C.** true **D.** true **E.** true

Chromosome abnormalities can essentially be divided into those involving numbers (polyploid, aneuploid) and those involving breakage or rearrangement (deletion, reciprocal translocations, ring chromosomes, Robertsonian translocation). See Paper 3 Question 1 for more details and examples.

Mitochondrial DNA deletions underlie Leber's optic atrophy, Leigh's necrotizing encephalopathy of childhood, and the mitochondrial myopathies. Mitochondria have their own genetic material in the form of a 16.6Kb, double stranded circular DNA molecule. Most mitochondrial proteins are encoded by the nuclear DNA however a small percentage are encoded by the mitochondrial DNA; for example 13 proteins involved in the respiratory chain required for oxidative phosphorylation. All mitochondrial DNA is inherited from generation to generation in a non-Mendelian manner, being transmitted only through the female line. This arises because the spermatozoal cytoplasm, including its mitochondria, is entirely lost at fertilization. Lebers optic atrophy shows such maternal transmission and is due to a mitochondrial mutation.

The main groups and clinical manifestations of diseases due to mitochondrial dysfunction:

Disease group	***Clinical manifestations***
Defects of fatty acid oxidation	Hypoglycaemia Hepatic dysfunction Cardiac failure Myopathy Sudden infant death

Respiratory chain disorders	Lactic acidosis Encephalopathy Hypotonia Poor feeding Failure to thrive Convulsions

Causes of some of the encephalopathies:

1. progressive external ophthalmoplegia (PEO)
2. Kearns Sayre syndrome
3. myoclonic epilepsy with ragged red fibres (MERRF)
4. mitochondrial encephalopathy, lactic acid, and stroke-like episodes (MELAS),
5. neurogenic weakness, ataxia, and retinitis pigmentosa

All of the above are due to primary single gene defects in mitochondrial DNA; some disorders due to gene defects in mitochondrial nuclear DNA have also been described.

Other examples:	type II diabetes plus deafness ?sideroblastic anaemia

Watts RWE. The inborn errors of metabolism: general aspects Oxford Textbook of Medicine. Oxford University Press.

Question 3

A. true **B.** false **C.** true **D.** true **E.** false

Some intracellular messengers:

Ca^{2+} ions	e.g. as a mediator for alpha adrenergic receptors
Protein kinase A	
Protein kinase C	
Cyclic AMP	e.g. as a mediator for beta adrenergic receptors
Diacylglycerol	
ATP	

Hormones are a good example of describing the various actions of intracellular messengers. Receptors for hormones are divided into membrane and nuclear receptors. Hormones that bind to membrane receptors act in combination with membrane-associated effector proteins to activate second messenger signalling pathways. The second messengers, whether cAMP, calcium, diacylglycerol, or others, stimulate a cascade of kinases, which then act upon target substrates on the membrane, in the cytoplasm, or in the nucleus.

Most of the cellular actions of nuclear receptors are mediated by changes in levels of mRNA which, in turn, alter levels of enzymes, hormones, or other proteins.

Jameson JL. Principles of hormone action.
Oxford Textbook of Medicine. Oxford University Press.

Question 4

A. false **B.** false **C.** false **D.** true **E.** false

See Paper 4 Question 4 for a discussion on Nitric Oxide.

To summarize Nitric Oxide

Synthesis:	from L-arginine
Half life:	seconds
Manufactured:	endothelium (principally in arteries)
Action:	potent vasodilator / inhibits platelet aggregation acts by increasing cGMP
Release:	possibly by shear stress along endothelium platelet derived mediators acetylcholine, bradykinin, substance P

Synthesis upregulated by Interleukin 1, TNF, ACE inhibitors

Vallance P Vascular endothelium, its physiology and pathophysiology.
Oxford Textbook of Medicine. Oxford University Press.

Question 5

A. false **B.** false **C.** false **D.** true **E.** false

Nerve	***Motor supply***
Median	thenar muscles abductor pollicis brevis flexor pollicis brevis (with ulnar nerve) opponens pollicis lumbricals to index and middle finger
Ulnar	flexor carpi ulnaris flexors of distal phalanx of ring / little fingers all intrinsic hand muscles certain of the thenar group: abductor pollicis, part of the flexor pollicis brevis
Radial	triceps brachioradialis supinator all extensors of the wrist, thumb and fingers

Scadding JW, Gibby J. Neurological disease
Oxford Textbook of Medicine. Oxford University Press.

Question 6

A. true **B.** false **C.** true **D.** true **E.** false

The outflow of the parasympathetic nervous system passes from the brain stem via nerves III, VII, IX and X. Some of the actions of this supply include:

constriction of the pupil
lacrimation
salivation
slowing of the heart
penile erection
emptying of the bladder

In addition to the cranial outflow there is also a sacral outflow via the pelvic splanchnic nerves (nervi erigentes), the source being the S2, S3 and S4 nerves.

Ger R, Abrahams P. Essentials of Clinical Anatomy
London Pitman Publishing

Question 7

A. true **B.** false **C.** true **D.** false **E.** false

See Paper 3 Question 7 for a discussion on Atrial Natriuretic Peptide.

Atrial Natriuretic Peptide

Synthesis:	in atrial wall
Release increased in:	atrial distension/stretch endothelin vasopressin catecholamines hypertension congestive cardiac failure
Actions:	acts on natriuretic peptide receptors A+B – by increasing cGMP low dose causes reduced peripheral resistance, lowers blood pressure higher doses increase peripheral resistance increase venous capacitance promotes natriuresis increases renal blood flow reduces renin and aldosterone concentration

Levin ER. Natriuretic Peptides
NEJM 1998 339: 5; 321–329

Question 8

A. false **B.** true **C.** false **D.** false **E.** true

Somatostatin is found widely throughout the central and peripheral nervous system, and in a variety of endocrine tissues. It exists in two forms (14 and 28 amino acids) in the gastrointestinal tract. Whilst secreted in specific endocrine cells in gastric and intestinal mucosa and D cells in the inner rim of the pancreatic islets it is also present in the enteric neural system. At least five somatostatin receptors have been isolated and cloned; type I occurs in the GI tract. Its principal action is to inhibit a number of hormones and it also inhibits a wide range of GI functions. It may also have an endocrine role.

Hormones inhibited by somatostatin: growth hormone, thyroid stimulating hormone, insulin, glucagon, pancreatic polypeptide, gastrin, secretin, gastric inhibitory polypeptide, motilin, enteroglucagon.

Physiological functions (inhibitory): lowers gastroesophageal sphincter contraction, gastric acid secretion, gastric emptying and secretions, absorption of nutrients, splanchnic blood flow, gallbladder contraction and secretions, pancreatic enzyme and bicarbonate secretion.

Hammond PJ et al. Hormones and the GI tract
Oxford Textbook of Medicine. Oxford University Press.

Question 9

A. true **B.** false **C.** true **D.** false **E.** false

Changes to blood pressure within an individual:

Exposure to pain
Stress (e.g. exposure to cold)
Exercise
Sexual intercourse
Lowest point: early in the morning
Maximum: on rising
In shift workers this circadian rhythm changes.

Loss of circadian rhythm changes in blood pressure are noted in immobile patients, autonomic dysfunction (e.g. diabetes), pre-eclampsia, cardiac transplantation and in some elderly hypertensives

Wilcken DEL. Clinical physiology of the normal heart
Oxford Textbook of Medicine. Oxford University Press.

Question 10

A. true **B.** false **C.** false **D.** true **E.** true

Growth hormone has been described as anabolic, lipolytic, and diabetogenic – its administration produces alterations in carbohydrate and lipid utilization. Upon administration to GH-deficient children it produces positive nitrogen balance, decreased urea production, redistributed body fat, and reduced carbohydrate utilization without development of diabetes. It has a direct effect on cells as well as actions mediated through insulin growth factor I (IGF-I) which acts through a negative homeostatic loop to reduce GH secretion.

Metabolic effects of growth hormone replacement:

Increased	lean body mass (anabolic effect)
	basal metabolic rate
	muscle strength, heart and exercise capacity
	bone mass and bone turnover
	glomerular filtration rate
	renal plasma flow
	plasma glucose (catabolic effect)
Reduced	plasma LDL-cholesterol

Thorner MO. Anterior pituitary disorders.
Oxford Textbook of Medicine. Oxford University Press.

Question 11

A. true **B.** false **C.** false **D.** true **E.** true

Causes of a metabolic acidosis:

Acute and chronic renal failure	
diabetic ketoacidosis	
lactic acidosis	
overdose of drugs	e.g. aspirin
	methanol
	ethylene glycol
	paraldehyde
renal tubular acidosis	
low albumin	
paraproteinaemia	
normal anion gap metabolic acidosis	

Cohen RD, Woods HF. Disturbances of acid-base homeostasis.
Oxford Textbook of Medicine. Oxford University Press.

Question 12

A. true **B.** true **C.** false **D.** true **E.** true

Causes of some primary immunodeficiencies

Antibody deficiency:	X linked agammaglobulinaemia common varied immunodeficiency thymoma with hypogammaglobulinaemia selective IgA deficiency selective IgG subclass deficiency transient hypogammaglobulinaemia of infancy
Selective T cell deficiency	thymic aplasia purine nucleoside phosphorylase deficiency T cell receptor defects
Mixed T and B cell defects	
severe	severe combined immunodeficiency e.g. X linked
moderate	e.g. Ataxic telangiectasia Wiskott Aldrich disease

Selective T cell deficiencies are very rare but provide information in the role of T cells in human infection and resistance to disease. Thymic aplasia (Di George syndrome) is associated in many cases with a structural defect of chromosome 22. Purine nucleoside phosphorylase (PNP) deficiency is characterised by T cell deficiency and the affected individual is vulnerable to severe Cytomegalovirus and varicella infection, autoimmune blood dyscrasias, lymphoma, and neurological disease with spasticity and muscle weakness.

T cell receptor defects are vanishingly rare. Most severe combined immunodeficiency disease (SCID) is due to rare inherited or spontaneous mutations of genes that influence the maturation of lymphocytes, particularly T cells. Infections are more severe than for the selective T cell deficiency probably because macrophage function is also affected.

Some causes of secondary immunodeficiencies

Lymphoreticular malignancy	CCL myeloma	
Drugs	steroids cyclophosphamide azathioprine cyclosporin	gold phenytoin penicillin sulphasalazine
Viruses	HIV rubella	

Metabolic/vitamin deficiency	vitamin A zinc selenium biotin renal and liver impairment
Hypercatabolism/increased loss	of immunoglobulins nephrotic syndrome protein losing enterophathy dystrophica myotonica

Lymphoid malignancies, immunosuppressive agents, and AIDS are common causes of severe immunodeficiency, while nutritional, metabolic disturbances and trauma have a less severe effect on the immune system. Recurrent pneumonia and bronchitis suggest antibody deficiency, whereas varicella zoster and herpes simplex reactivation, oral candidiasis, and rapid growth of skin warts are often early indications of a defect in cellular immunity.

McMichael AJ. Principles of Immunology
Oxford Textbook of Medicine. Oxford University Press.

Question 13

A. true **B.** true **C.** true **D.** true **E.** false

One group of autoantibodies that has received much attention as a marker for inflammatory disease is the antineutrophil cytoplasmic autoantibody (cANCA). Specific for proteinase 3 found in primary lysosomes, these antibodies are markers for Wegener's granulomatosis, crescentic nephritides and vasculitis.

Common antibodies seen in connective tissue disease:

Anti-dsDNA	SLE
Anti-Sm	SLE
Anti-U1RNP	SLE/overlap syndrome (MCTD)
Anti-Ro	SLE/Sjogrens
Anti-La	SLE/Sjogrens
Anticentromere	limited cutaneous scleroderma (CREST)
Anti-Scl-70	diffuse cutaneous scleroderma
Anti-Jo-1	polymyositis, lung involvement
cANCA	Wegener's granulomatosis
pANCA	microscopic PAN, other vasculitides also seen in ulcerative colitis
anticardiolipin	SLE with thrombosis, miscarriages etc

Black CM, Scott DGI. Rheumatology – introduction
Oxford Textbook of Medicine. Oxford University Press.

Question 14

A. true **B.** false **C.** true **D.** false **E.** true

Infectious mononucleosis presents in 75% of cases with a sore throat, 15% of cases as a hepatitis, and in 10% of cases simply as a fever. The infection is usually asymptomatic in young children but is increasingly symptomatic with age, usually presenting as typical glandular fever in adolescents and young adults. The causative agent, Epstein-Barr virus, is a dsDNA herpesvirus that codes for 100–200 proteins. Antibodies to the Epstein-Barr nuclear antigen (EBNA) and the early antigen (EA) appear initially but are transient. IgM and IgG antibody to capsid antigens subsequently appear with IgG anti-capsid antibody persisting for life. The virus infects B lymphocytes which then cause T-cell activation and multiplication. These give rise to the atypical mononuclear cells that are present in the peripheral blood stream. There is usually a 6–8 week incubation period followed by the development of fever, sore throat, and widespread tender lymphadenopathy. Gross tonsillar and pharyngeal swelling can develop which can compromise the airway. Splenomegaly, a mild hepatitis and a maculopapular rash are relatively common. The later occurs in over 90% of cases who are given ampicillin erroneously for a sore throat.

Rarer complications include thrombocytopenia, haemolytic anaemia, myocarditis, meningitis, encephalitis, mononeuritis, mesenteric adenitis, splenic rupture and Guillain-Barré syndrome. A post-infectious fatigue may develop that resolves over 3–6 months.

Early diagnosis before the appearance of IgM anti-EBV antibody is by the Paul-Bunnell test. This detects heterophile antibodies which agglutinate horse and sheep red blood cells. Causes of a false positive result include viral hepatitis, Hodgkin's lymphoma, and leukaemia.

There is no specific treatment though occasionally steroids may be necessary if neurological complications occur.

Epstein MA, Crawford DH. The Epstein-Barr Virus
Ledingham JGG, Warrell DA. Concise Oxford Textbook of Medicine. 2000. Oxford University Press.

Question 15

A. false **B.** false **C.** false **D.** true **E.** false

Giardia lamblia (intestinalis) is a protozoa ingested in cyst form that develops into a motile trophozoite in the upper small intestine. It is spread by the oro-faecal route and waterborne transmission. The infection occurs world-wide though is much commoner in developing countries with poor sanitation. It can cause a variety of mucosal appearances in the small intestine ranging from normal, through infiltrative lesions, to a flat mucosa. However it is not a common cause of total villous atrophy. Clinically the picture varies from asymptomatic disease to acute or chronic diarrhoea with malabsorption. The incubation period ranges from 1 to 6 weeks. Symptoms include nausea, anorexia, weight loss, abdominal pain, loose bulky stools, steatorrhoea, belching, flatulence, and borborygmi. Haematochezia is unusual and alternative diagnoses should be considered. Diagnosis is usually made by cyst identification from a stool sample. Three stool samples should be sent as cysts are shed intermittently. In experienced hands this has a sensitivity approaching 90%. The diagnosis can also be made from a duodenal aspirate or biopsies.

Treatment is with metronidazole for 3 days or tinidazole as a single dose.

Katelaris P, Farthing MJG. Tropical and infective diseases of the gastrointestinal tract and liver. Shearman DJC, Finlayson NDC et al. Diseases of the Gastrointestinal Tract and Liver. 3rd Ed. 1997 Churchill Livingstone. London.

Question 16

A. false **B.** true **C.** false **D.** true **E.** true

A prion is a protein that occurs in normal brain tissue. Its function is unknown and knockout animal models appear to function normally. The term prion was initially coined to represent the proteinaceous infectious agent found to cause scrapie in sheep.

There are several prion related diseases in humans of which Creutzfeldt-Jacob disease is the most common and best known. Prion diseases arise following a conformational change in normal soluble prion protein to an insoluble form. The insoluble form is not metabolized and thus accumulates in cells eventually causing cell death. It is resistant to proteinases and can withstand high temperatures. This change in the conformation of prion protein can be acquired spontaneously, occur in a hereditary fashion due to a gene mutation, or be transmitted in an infectious manner. Unlike other infectious agents, no genetic material is involved in transmission of disease which occurs from the abnormal protein complexing with a normal prion protein in the host inducing conformational change. Transmission of the disease can occur through direct inoculation of the abnormal protein or through ingestion following which the latent or incubation period of the disease is longer.

Fleminger S, Curtis D. Prion diseases.
Br J Psych 1997 170(2): 103–105

Question 17

A. true **B.** false **C.** false **D.** true **E.** true

Plasmodium falciparum is the only malarial parasite that causes severe complicated disease. It is distinct from the other species in that it expresses novel proteins on the surface of infected red blood cells that cause sequestration of the blood cells in tissues such as brain, lung, and bone marrow. The parasite enters the host blood in the sporozoite form through the bite of a female anopheline mosquito. The sporozoite then multiplies in the liver producing merozoites which are released back into the circulation where they penetrate red blood cells. They then grow as trophozoites in the red blood cells until dividing again into multiple merozoites, lysing the red blood cell and re-entering the circulation. P. falciparum does not form hypnozoites in the liver and thus only recurs if inadequately treated initially. The incubation period is usually 1–2 weeks but can be prolonged, especially following chemoprophylaxis with some cases presenting 3–12 months after leaving an endemic area. Typical symptoms include fever (classically tertian), rigors, anorexia, headache, myalgia, nausea, vomiting and diarrhoea. Anaemia, jaundice and hepatosplenomegaly often occur.

Complications include cerebral malaria with encephalopathy, fitting and coma, severe anaemia and DIC, hypoglycaemia, renal failure, and haemoglobinuria (blackwater fever). Autoimmune anaemia and thrombocytopenia may occur. Parasitaemia of >4% is associated with a high risk of complicated disease. Treatment of uncomplicated disease is with oral quinine for 7 days unless the infection is from a known area of low chloroquine resistance in which case chloroquine can be used. A single dose of sulfadoxine and pyrimethamine, or mefloquine, or a five day course of doxycycline should be given after the first few days of treatment.

Treatment of severe disease is with intravenous quinine and appropriate management of complications. Intravenous quinine may cause hypoglycaemia and tinnitus.

Bradley D, Newbold CI, Warrell DA. Malaria
Oxford Textbook of Medicine. Oxford University Press.

Question 18

A. false **B.** true **C.** true **D.** true **E.** false

Von Willebrand's disease is inherited in an autosomal dominant manner. The gene defect has been located on chromosome 12. It affects both sexes and is the commonest inherited coagulopathy in the UK. There is a quantitative or qualitative abnormality of von Willebrand's factor (vWF).

vWF has 2 functions:

1. It acts as a carrier protein for factor VIIIC protecting it from breakdown
2. It is involved in platelet aggregation and adhesion.

There more than 20 different subtypes of the disease.

There is a varied clinical picture. Symptoms may be intermittent and relate to platelet dysfunction such as epistaxis, bruising etc. It is very rare to have a haemarthrosis. The platelet count is normal as is the PT. The APTT or PTTK is increased. The bleeding time is increased. The addition of ristocetin to plasma of a patient does not cause platelet aggregation.

Management includes:

1. Avoidance of aspirin and NSAIDs
2. Tranexamic acid
3. DDAVP in some cases
4. Fresh frozen plasma, (they do not need platelets).

Disorders of bleeding time:

Mild coagulopathy:	vWF Mild haemophilia Factor XII deficiency Bernard Soulier syndrome

Platelet dysfunction:	Aspirin ingestion Dysproteinemia (esp. IgA) Inherited platelet defect Platelet factor III deficiency Grey platelet syndrome Glanzmann's thrombasthenia Hereditary afibrinogenaemia
Others	Vascular disorders - Hereditary haemorrhagic telangiectasia - Vasculitis, scurvy Hereditary connective tissue disorders - Ehlers-Danlos syndrome - Osteogenesis imperfecta - pseudoxanthoma elasticum - Marfan's syndrome

Epstein RJ. Medicine for Examinations
Churchill Livingstone 1996

Question 19

A. false **B.** true **C.** true **D.** false **E.** false

Iron is usually in plentiful supply in the western diet. A normal diet usually contains around 15mg/day. 5–10% of dietary iron is absorbed. Absorption occurs in the duodenum and upper jejunum. It is better absorbed in the Ferrous than the Ferric form. This is aided by gastric acid and vitamin C.

The total body store is around 4g. 1mg/day is lost in urine, sweat and cells shed from the skin and GI tract. Menstrual loss is around 20mg/month.

Iron is stored as ferritin. Transferrin is a carrier protein for iron.

Serum iron levels are often reduced in inflammatory disease including inflammatory bowel disease.

Factors influencing iron absorption

Increase	***Decrease***
Dietary factors	
Increased haem iron	Decreased haem iron
Increased meat	Decreased meat
Luminal factors	
Acid pH (e.g. gastric HCl)	Alkalis (e.g. pancreatic secretions)
Soluble iron complexes with e.g.:	Insoluble iron complexes with e.g.:
Ascorbic acid	Phytates
Sugars	Phosphates

Amino acids Meat factor	Tea (tannates) Bran
Systemic factors	
Reduced iron stores	Increased iron stores
Increased erythropoiesis (especially in dyserythropoietic anaemias)	Decreased erythropoiesis
Hypoxia	Inflammatory disorders

Factors influencing serum iron, total iron binding capacity (TIBC), and ferritin measurements

Measurement	***Increase***	***Decrease***
Serum iron	Fe overload Liver disease Decreased erythropoiesis (e.g. aplastic anaemia) Haemolysis/dyserythropoiesis (e.g. pernicious anaemia)	Fe deficiency Infection/inflammation
Serum TIBC	Iron deficiency Pregnancy Oral contraceptive	Iron overload Infection/inflammation Protein loss/malnutrition
Serum ferritin	Iron overload Liver disease Infection/inflammation Malignancy Haemolytic anaemia Hyperthyroidism Spleen or bone marrow infarction	Iron deficiency

Pippard MJ. Iron metabolism and its disorders
Oxford Textbook of Medicine. Oxford University Press.

Question 20

A. true **B.** true **C.** false **D.** false **E.** false

Megaloblastic erythropoiesis due to folic acid deficiency some causes:

1.	Decreased intake	poverty old age alcoholics
2.	Increased requirements	pregnancy increased cell turnover such as in haemolysis or renal dialysis

3.	Malabsorption	coeliac disease Crohn' s disease tropical sprue
4.	Drugs	phenytoin nitrofurantoin oral contraceptive pill barbiturates
5.	Antifolate drugs	methotrexate trimethoprim pentamidine
6.	Alcohol	poor nutrition and direct depressant effect.

Epstein RJ. Medicine for Examinations
Churchill Livingstone 1996

Question 21

A. false **B.** true **C.** true **D.** true **E.** false

Predisposing factors to deep venous thrombosis include

Post operative (eg. increased risk in up to 50% of orthopaedic patients)
Immobility for more than 3–4 days
Age over 40 years
Previous deep vein thrombosis and or embolism
Sepsis
malignancy
pregnancy/puerperium
oral contraceptive pill
Nephrotic syndrome

Rare conditions: paroxysmal nocturnal haemoglobinuria, homocystinuria and Behçet's disease.

It is important to screen for deficiencies in protein c, protein s, antithrombin III, lupus anticoagulant, factor V lieden and resistance to activated protein C.

Controversial: long car journeys, cigarette smoking and long haul air travel (due to dehydration and alcohol consumption) it is likely that the latter subject will be clarified with current trials in the next 2–3 years.

Weatherall DJ. Haematology: introduction
Oxford Textbook of Medicine. Oxford University Press.

Paper 5 Answers

Question 22

A. false **B.** false **C.** false **D.** true **E.** true

Salbutamol causes the intracellular movement of potassium and hence causes hypokalaemia. This can be used therapeutically in the correction of hyperkalaemia. Insulin also causes the intracellular movement of potassium. The emergency treatment of hyperkalaemia is calcium gluconate to stabilize the myocardium, followed by the administration of 10 IU of Actrapid and 50mls of 50% dextrose. This may only buy time for 2–3 hours: long enough to allow correction of the underlying abnormality and/or arrange haemodialysis. The correction of megaloblastic anaemia can cause hypokalaemia by redistribution of potassium.

Other drugs causing hypokalaemia include:

thiazide diuretics
loop diuretics
corticosteroids – by increased renal excretion
carbenoxolone
laxative abuse

Nephrotoxic drugs such as amino glycosides or amphotericin may cause renal tubular damage and hypokalaemia

Burton JL, Healey CJ. Aids to Postgraduate Medicine
Sixth Edition, Churchill Livingstone 1994

Question 23

A. false **B.** false **C.** true **D.** true **E.** false

Sodium valproate is used in the treatment of partial seizures, petit mal epilepsy and generalized absences. It increases GABA levels by preventing its breakdown and uptake into cells. It is well absorbed orally, metabolized by the liver and 90% is protein bound. The half-life is 8–12 hours and so multiple daily dosing is required. Plasma concentrations are not helpful and are not usually monitored. It is the anticonvulsant of choice in Acute Intermittent Porphyria.

Side effects of sodium valproate include

nausea
transient hair loss – regrowth is curly
thrombocytopenia
drug induced hepatitis
weight gain through increased appetite
ataxia and tremor

pancreatitis
Neural tube defects when given in the 1st trimester

Some commonly used drugs that are known to be teratogenic

Drug	***Abnormality***
Phenytoin	Craniofacial
Carbamazepine	Limb/fingernail Cardiac
Sodium valproate	Neural tube
Phenobarbitone	Cleft palate
Warfarin	Chondrodysplasia punctata Koala bear facies CNS anomalies
Lithium	Cardiac (Ebstein complex), cretinism
Danazol	Virilization of female fetus
Retinoids	Multiple

Lima JM. The new drugs and the strategies to manage epilepsy Curr.Pharm.Des 2000 6: 8; 873–878

Question 24

A. true **B.** true **C.** true **D.** false **E.** false

Chloroquine is used in the chemoprophylaxis and treatment of malaria but there is increasing resistance worldwide. It is also used in the treatment of rheumatoid arthritis and SLE. Although usually very well tolerated the side effects of chloroquine include:

Visual disturbances
Depigmentation or hair loss
Headaches
Convulsions
Bone marrow suppression
Ototoxicity
Keratopathy
GI disturbances but not GI bleeds
Corneal opacities – long term usage normally
Stevens-Johnson syndrome.

Retinal degeneration – it used to be recommended that patients on chloroquine or hydroxychloroquine have annual ophthalmological review: this is no longer recommended, but the elderly should have a base line review before initiation of treatment.

Jones SK. Ocular toxicity and hydroxychloroquine: guidelines for screening British Journal of Dermatology 1999 140(1): 3–7

Question 25

A. true **B.** true **C.** false **D.** true **E.** true

Major side effects of the oral contraceptive pill (OCP):

Increased risk of venous thromboembolic disease, especially in smokers. The risk increases with age. The risk of thromboembolism in women not taking the OCP is 5/100,000. The risk if on the oral contraceptive is 15–25/100,000. The risk in pregnancy is 60/100,000

Increased risk of MI and CVA

Hypertension

There is a slight increase risk of breast cancer with the combined OCP. The risk is related to the age at which the OCP is stopped. The risk decreases in the 10 years after cessation of treatment such that by 10 years there is no excess risk. It should be used with caution in patients with a family history of breast carcinoma.

Other side effects include

- headaches and may worsen migraines
- mood swings
- breast tenderness
- irregular bleeding
- cholestatic jaundice
- depression
- fluid retention
- chorea
- skin reactions
- benign intracranial hypotension
- hepatic adenomas

British National Formulary
BMA and Royal Pharmaceutical Society of Great Britain

Vandenbroucke JP. Oral contraceptives and the risk of venous thrombosis NEJM 2001 344: 20; 1527–1535

Question 26

A. false **B.** true **C.** true **D.** true **E.** true

Hyperprolactinaemia is associated with

- galactorrhea
- oligo/amenorrhea
- decreased libido
- decreased potency
- delayed puberty

subfertility
headaches and visual field defects can occur if the cause is a pituitary tumour.

Treatment is with a dopamine agonist such as bromocriptine. This will correct the symptoms. It may lead to shrinkage of a tumour but this is NOT characteristic

Gynaecomastia denotes the enlargement of the male breast caused by proliferation of the glandular tissue. The most important differential diagnosis is carcinoma of the male breast. Whilst gynaecomastia is common in Klinefelter's syndrome it is distinct from all other causes as Klinefelter patients have a 16 times greater risk of carcinoma of the breast. Conservative medical treatment is unlikely to be successful if the condition has lasted over 12 months due to fibrotic tissue. It is rare in hyperprolactinaemia.

Causes of gynaecomastia:	Physiological & Pathological
Testosterone deficiency	Klinefelter's syndrome Viral orchitis (eg mumps) Trauma Neurological eg myotonica dystrophica spinal cord lesions African trypanosomiasis
Increased oestrogen production	Leydig and Sertoli cell tumours true hermaphroditism congenital adrenal hyperplasia adrenal carcinoma
Liver disease	increased plasma/urine excretion of oestrogen reduced secretion of testosterone (gonadal atrophy) decreased hepatic extraction of androstenedione
Malnutrition/starvation	
Drugs	oestrogen enhancers eg HCG, clomiphene testosterone inhibitors eg. cyproterone acetate, flutamide, cimetidine diuretics: principally spironolactone cannabis
Malignancy	carcinoma of the lung: large cell
Neurological	trinucleotide repeats: principally Kennedy's syndrome
POEMS syndrome	
Infections	leprosy

Turner HE. Gynaecomastia
Medicine 1997 25: 5; 41–43

Bevan JS. Prolactin Disorders
Medicine1997 25: 4; 6–8

Question 27

A. false **B.** true **C.** true **D.** true **E.** true

3,4-methylenedioxymethamphetamine (MDMA, or ecstasy) is a semi synthetic hallucinogenic drug. It has a brief duration of action of around 4–6 hours.

Recognized features include:

tachycardias
hyperpyrexia
tonic movements
convulsions
coagulopathy
rhabdomyolysis
renal failure
liver failure
ARDS

Milroy CM. Ten years of ecstasy
Royal Society of Medicine 1999 92(2): 68–72

Question 28

A. false **B.** false **C.** true **D.** false **E.** true

The Chi squared test should only be done on actual numbers not proportions or percentages. It is used to test for differences between 2 independently derived proportions. If a table is constructed in this example it would be a 2 by 2 table. The degree of freedom is the product of the number of columns-1 × number of rows –1. So in this case there is one degree of freedom.

The calculated value of chi squared must be converted into a probability using tables. Congenital heart disease would be a confounding variable and lead to error. A confounding variable is a factor (not being studied) that is different between the populations and that would affect the outcome being studied.

Driscoll P et al. Statistics 5: An introduction to estimation 2. Starting from Z to t. J Accid Emerg Med 2001 18: 65–70

Question 29

A. true **B.** true **C.** false **D.** false **E.** true

See Paper 1 Question 31 for a discussion on SLE.

Question 30

A. false **B.** false **C.** false **D.** true **E.** true

Polymyalgia rheumatica (PMR) is common. The annual incidence is around 20/100,000. Most patients are 60–70 years old, but 1/3 of patients are under 60. Women are affected 3 times more often than men. The symptoms are of limb girdle pain and their onset may be acute or insidious. The condition may be associated with early morning stiffness. The ESR is normally raised and the LFT's may be abnormal. It can be associated with a fever, malaise and weight loss. There is muscle tenderness. On commencing treatment the response to corticosteroids is dramatic. If the response is delayed then an alternative diagnosis must be considered. It can occur with giant cell/cranial arteritis and if this is suspected treatment should not be withheld until the diagnosis is biopsy proven as delay can lead to blindness. The latest ophthalmic advice is that changes can still be seen on biopsy even 2 weeks after starting steroids.

Mowat AG. Polymyalgia rheumatica and giant cell arteritis
Oxford Textbook of Medicine. Oxford University Press

Question 31

A. false **B.** false **C.** false **D.** true **E.** false

Reiter's syndrome consists of a triad of non specific urethritis, conjunctivitis and seronegative arthritis. It occurs following either a dysenteric illness or a sexually transmitted disease. It affects males more than females. 75% are HLA B27 positive. The arthritis usually begins 1–3 weeks after an infection. It does not respond to treatment of the infection.

Other features include

- oral ulceration
- circinate balanitis
- keratoderma blenorrhagica
- iritis

plantar fascitis
sacroiliitis
fever and/or weight loss

More rarely there may be involvement of the:

cardiac system – pericarditis, aortitis or conduction defects
respiratory system – pleurisy, pulmonary infiltrates
CNS – peripheral neuropathy or meningoencephalitis.

70–75% resolve with no recurrence.
20–25% resolve but then recur. This is more likely in HLA B27 positive patients.
<5% develop chronic problems, again more in the HLA B27 positive group.

Treatment is with NSAIDs. Steroids are used in the presence of systemic symptoms. If the condition becomes chronic they may require a disease modifying agent of rheumatological disease (DMARD)

Keat A Post-infective arthritides
Medicine 1998 26: 6; 43–46

Question 32

A. false **B.** true **C.** true **D.** true **E.** false

(For our convenience this question is in the gastroenterology section but as with many of the college questions there is a single stem that acts to test your knowledge of lists across many different subjects).

Hepatitis A in the young is usually a mild disease and is anicteric. It may cause a severe, fulminant hepatitis, but this is generally in the middle aged onwards. It does not cause chronic hepatitis or cirrhosis. 2) Late effects of ALL treatment include structural damage to the central nervous system, endocrine abnormalities and secondary malignancies (the latter occurring in around 8% of survivors, and involve haematological malignancies, AML and non-Hodgkin's lymphomas). 3) In phenylketonuria strict dietary control of phenylalanine is necessary to prevent brain damage, and although this is often relaxed later on, some patients are more difficult to control than others, and many patients still develop demyelination in later life despite apparently remaining on a diet. Subtle psychological changes may occur even in well-controlled patients who are otherwise normal on IQ and developmental tests. 4) Whilst coarctation may be a sporadic occurence, remember for the purposes of the exam that it is also a feature of both Noonan's and Turner's syndrome. Although the perioperative mortality for elective surgery is low, patients require careful medical follow-up as many encounter significant morbidity and mortality in later life. Long-term prognosis is inversely related to the extent and duration of preoperative hypertension. Hypertension is common after repair.

Minimal change nephropathy rarely causes long-term sequelae, particularly in children.

Bobby JJ et al. Operative survival and 40 year follow-up of surgical repair of aortic coarctation. British Heart Journal 1991 65: 271–276

Brenton DP. Inborn errors of amino acid and organic acid metabolism. In Weatherall DJ, Ledingham JGG, Warrell DA, eds. Oxford Textbook of Medicine, Oxford: Oxford University Press, 1996.

Question 33

A. false **B.** false **C.** true **D.** true **E.** false

Obstruction to the right outflow tract can occur at several levels causing pulmonary stenosis. Pulmonary artery stenosis causing supravalvular stenosis occurs in Williams syndrome and following intrauterine rubella. (Williams syndrome: elf like facies, hypercalcaemia, supravalvular aortic and pulmonary stenosis).

Pulmonary valve stenosis most commonly occurs as an isolated congenital abnormality though also occurs in Noonan's syndrome, Fallot's tetrology, congenital rubella, following surgery, and in carcinoid syndrome.

Subvalvular infundibular stenosis occurs due to hypertrophied muscle bands below the pulmonary valve and is usually associated with a VSD.

Clinical signs associated with pulmonary stenosis include giant a wave in JVP, right ventricular hypertrophy, ejection systolic click and murmur, widely split 2nd heart sound which increases on inspiration, clubbing and peripheral cyanosis.

For a discussion on atrial septal defects see Paper 1 Question 32.

Murmurs heard in ASD

1. pulmonary flow murmur
2. tricuspid flow murmur
3. pulmonary regurgitation (Graham Steel murmur of pulmonary hypertension)

Other features of an ASD

CXR:	pulmonary plethora, RV enlargement
ECG:	RAD + incomplete RBBB (secundum)
	LAD + complete RBBB (primum)
	long pr (first degree heart block)
Echo:	paradoxical septal motion
	RV enlargement
	visualization of the shunt using contrast (bubbles are seen if the shunt is patent)
catheterization:	shunt size pulmonary hypertension

Swanton RH. Cardiology 4th Ed. 1998. Blackwell Scientific Publications Ltd. Oxford

Question 34

A. false **B.** true **C.** false **D.** false **E.** false

Following DC cardioversion for atrial fibrillation only 10–30% of cases remain in sinus rythmn at 1year. Factors associated with this are young age, recent onset AF (generally <3 months), and a structurally normal heart.

Pre-treatment with antiarrymthmics such as amiodarone improve the conversion rate to and maintenance of sinus rythmn. However the optimum drug, timing, and dose remain unknown.

Ledingham JGG, Warrell DA. Concise Oxford Textbook of Medicine. 2000 Oxford University Press. Oxford.

Question 35

A. false **B.** true **C.** false **D.** false **E.** true

Jugular venous pulse waveform

'a' wave: atrial systole

giant 'a' wave: pulmonary stenosis, pulmonary hypertension, tricuspid stenosis

Cannon wave: atrial systole against closed tricuspid valve
junctional tachycardia, complete heart block, ventricular extrasystole

'a' wave lost in atrial fibrillation

'x' descent fall in atrial pressure during ventricular systole
prominent in pericardial constriction
prominent in pericardial tamponade

'v' wave: atrial filling against closed tricuspid valve

'y' descent: opening of tricuspid valve
prominent in pericardial constriction

's' wave is fusion of 'x' descent and 'v' wave in tricuspid regurgitation also known as giant 'a' wave.

Swanton RH. Cardiology 4th Ed. 1998. Blackwell Scientific Publications Ltd. Oxford

Question 36

A. true **B.** false **C.** false **D.** true **E.** true

Neurological sequelae of HIV infection.

HIV encephalopathy or dementia occurs in up to 10% of cases due to direct infection of the nervous system. It initially presents with gradual intellectual deterioration, mood changes, and inability to concentrate. The course is progressive and ultimately results in mutism, incontinence, and severe motor dysfunction. Physical signs include motor weakness, incoordination, hyper-reflexia, and extensor plantars. Antiretroviral therapy delays progression of the dementia.

Cerebral toxoplasmosis occurs in patients when the CD4 count <200. Patients develop fever, headache, focal neurological signs and typically have multiple ring enhancing lesions on CT or MRI. Treatment is with sulfadiazine and pyrimethamine.

Cryptococcal meningitis usually presents subacutely with constitutional malaise, fever, headache, and meningism. Diagnosis is by identifying cryptococci in the CSF by India ink staining. The CSF white cell count can be normal or only mildly raised and the CSF protein and glucose are often normal. Treatment is with fluconazole for mild illness or amphotericin B for severe illness plus or minus flucytosine. Secondary prophylaxis with an antifungal agent is necessary following treatment.

Progressive multifocal leucoencephalopathy (PML) is due to JC virus infection and occurs in advanced AIDS. It is a demyelinating illness that presents with focal neurological signs, ataxia, or personality changes. Diagnosis is made by recognizing the typical features on MRI. There is no specific treatment though combination antiretroviral therapy can slow and even reverse progression.

CMV encephalitis occurs in advanced AIDS with confusion, dementia, reduced conscious level, and convulsions. Diagnosis is by detecting CMV in the CSF and treatment is with ganciclovir or sodium foscarnet.

Non-Hodgkin's lymphoma arises in up to 10% of patients with HIV with the CNS being commonly affected. Median survival is about 3 months with neither radiotherapy or chemotherapy being of much benefit. Primary brain tumours are no more common than in the general population.

HIV can also cause vascular myelopathy, peripheral neuropathy, demylinating polyneuropathy, and autonomic neuropathy.

Ledingham JGG, Warrell DA. Concise Oxford Textbook of Medicine. 2000 Oxford University Press. Oxford.

Question 37

A. true **B.** false **C.** false **D.** true **E.** false

Dystrophia myotonica is the most common muscular dystrophy in the U.K. with an incidence of 1:8,000. It is inherited in an autosomal dominant manner and usually becomes apparent during adolescence or early adulthood.

The classical features are myotonia (delayed muscle relaxation), ptosis, weakness and wasting of facial and distal limb muscles, frontal balding, cataracts, cardiomyopathy and conduction defects, adrenal atrophy, testicular atrophy, infertility, hyperinsulinaemia or diabetes, and a low I.Q.

Diagnosis is usually based upon typical clinical features, family history, and compatible findings on EMG and muscle biopsy. More recently the genetic defect has been identified as a trinucleotide repeat on chromosome 19. Amplification of the defect gives rise to genetic anticipation where an increased number of trinucleotide repeats occurs in successive generations increasing disease severity.

Treatment is symptomatic with the myotonia responding to phenytoin, carbamazepine or acetazolamide.

Meola G. Myotonic Dystrophies
Current Opinion in Neurology 2000 13(5): 519–525

Question 38

A. false **B.** true **C.** false **D.** true **E.** false

Carotid artery stenosis may give rise to transient ischaemic attacks through embolization or low blood flow. TIAs related to low flow are usually brief, repetitive attacks that often herald strokes in the distribution of the internal carotid artery. Embolic TIAs are usually single and more prolonged events. They most commonly affect the middle cerebral artery which may give rise to contralateral hemiparesis, hemisensory loss, and homonymous hemianopia. Amaurosis fugax is transient monocular blindness caused by an embolus to the ophthalmic artery. A carotid bruit indicates carotid stenosis and may act as a marker of non-focal advanced atherosclerosis. In the Framingham study the finding of a carotid bruit was associated with a doubling of the risk of stroke though this often occurred in a vascular territory different to that of the bruit. 75% of patients with a carotid bruit have moderate to severe carotid stenosis though bruits are also absent in 1/3rd of cases with a high-grade stenosis.

Wolf PA et al. Asymptomatic carotid bruit and risk of stroke.
The Framingham study.
JAMA 1981 245: 1442

Inzitari D et al. The causes and risk of Stroke in patients with Asymptomatic Internal Carotid Artery Stenosis. NEJM 2000 342: 23; 1693–1701 and Editorial: Kistler JP et al. Carotid Artery Stenosis Revisited NEJM 2000 342: 23; 1743–1745

Question 39

A. true **B.** true **C.** true **D.** false **E.** true

Causes of a lower seizure threshold include

Infection
Head injury
Photosensitivity
Strobe lights
Sleep deprivation
Alcohol withdrawal
Electrolyte imbalance

Stress
Hormonal changes associated with the menstrual cycle
Withdrawal of anti-epileptic drugs

For a comprehensive review of the management of epilepsy see references below.

Brodie MJ et al. Management of epilepsy in adolescents and adults. The Lancet. 2000 356: 323–329

Browne TR, Holmes GL. Epilepsy
NEJM 2001 344: 15; 1145–1151

Question 40

A. false **B.** true **C.** true **D.** false **E.** false

Some of these questions have been answered in Paper 1 Question 40 and Paper 4 Question 43. Osteoporosis and ultimately dorsal kyphosis do occur. Parotid swelling occurs as a consequence of repeated vomiting. Finger clubbing does not occur, and thyroid hormones are usually low or normal.

Investigating anorexia nervosa:

elevated urea on biochemistry profile
abnormal liver function tests
sick euthyroid
elevated cortisol, growth hormone, cholesterol and reduced somatomedin C
multifollicular cystic ovaries on pelvic ultrasound
ECG abnormalities including prolonged QT

Stoving RK. Hangaard J. Hansen-Nord M. Hagen C. A review of endocrine changes in anorexia nervosa. Journal of Psychiatric Research 1999 . 33(2):139–152

Question 41

A. false **B.** true **C.** false **D.** false **E.** true

This question has been dealt with in Paper 4 Question 40.

Question 42

A. true **B.** false **C.** true **D.** false **E.** true

Some psychological, psychiatric and personality disorders are inter-dependent; certain depressive, anxious or inadequate people isolate themselves, drink for relief and become dependent.

Pathological jealousy and persecutory delusions occur in alcoholism, although non-delusional suspiciousness of the patients partners or friends is more common.

Alcoholic hallucinosis occurs in heavy drinkers. Voices may become suddenly apparent in consciousness or a mild delirious state lasting a day or so ushers in the hallucinosis. The patient believes the voices to come from above his or her head and they talk about him in the third person in a disparaging manner.

Illusions and delusional perception of sensory stimuli, and occasionally visual hallucinations occur, particularly at night. Classically Lilliputian hallucinations; lots of little men, or spiders occur.

Hallucinosis lasts longer than delirium tremens, which usually is over in a week. Half the patients recover in a month, although some do not recover within 6 months and remain chronic with intellectual impairment.

Neuropsychiatric manifestations of alcoholism:

1. Epilepsy, which may complicate acute alcohol intoxication, chronic heavy alcohol ingestion, alcohol withdrawal, subdural haematoma
2. Withdrawal related such as tremulousness, agitation, delirium tremens
3. Toxic neuronal degeneration secondary to cerebral atrophy or central pontine myelinolysis (often precipitated by hypertonic saline or lactulose)
4. Nutritional related (reduced vitamin intake) such as Wernicke's encephalopathy, Korsakoff's psychosis, pellagra, neuropathy (typically painful), tobacco alcohol amblyopia

Mark Ashworth and Claire Gerada. ABC of mental health. Addiction and dependence II: Alcohol. BMJ 1997 315: 358–360.

Question 43

A. true **B.** false **C.** false **D.** true **E.** true

Persecutory or paranoid delusions are common in schizophrenia, paraphrenia, depressive psychosis and some organic states such as alcoholism. Amphetamines and cocaine use commonly cause persecutory delusions. Generally affective disorders or so-called neuroses, and obsessional states do not cause psychotic symptoms such as delusional thought; in these situations other diagnoses should be considered if persecutory disorders are prominent. Depressive neurosis as a term to describe mild dementia without psychosis is not really used in modern psychiatry.

Turner T. ABC of mental health: Schizophrenia. BMJ 1997 315: 108–111

Question 44

A. false **B.** false **C.** true **D.** true **E.** true

Although in the ideal situation all alveolar-capillary units have equal matching of ventilation and perfusion; i.e. the average ventilation/perfusion ratio for the whole lung at rest is one, in the normal individual some ventilation/perfusion mismatching is present, due to the gradients of blood flow and ventilation between the bases and apices.

The distribution of blood volume and the distribution of blood flow when standing is much higher in the base than the apex. Ventilation increases from top to bottom of the lungs, although less steeply than blood flow. The reasons for this are thought to be both anchorage of blood vessels at the hilum and gravitational effects. Ventilation/perfusion ratios therefore tend to be higher in the bases of the apices of the lungs.

Arterial hypoxaemia in left ventricular failure is due to ventilation/perfusion mismatching. Hypercapnia, which is seen in a small proportion of cases, may be the result of further, severe, ventilation/perfusion imbalance.

In lobar pneumonia the consolidated lobe is perfused but not ventilated as it is filled with pus. This thus forms a physiological right to left shunt, with blood passing through the diseased lung without being oxygenated.

Weinberger SE, Drazen JM. Disturbances of respiratory function. In Isselbacher KJ, Braunwald E, Wilson JD et al., eds. Harrisons Principles of Internal Medicine, 13th Edition. New York: McGraw-Hill, 1994.

Question 45

A. true **B.** true **C.** false **D.** false **E.** false

Although inexperienced junior doctors and nurses hesitate to give high-flow oxygen in acute severe asthma, these patients have not lost their sensitivity to carbon dioxide and do not depend on hypoxic drive. In fact giving low concentration to a patient in this situation would probably be considered grossly negligent. Equally a man of 25 is unlikely to develop heart failure. The hyperventilation will exacerbate his dehydration, and he may well become hypotensive as a result.

Benzodiazepines and opiates are generally contraindicated, as these can blunt the respiratory drive, cause confusion if patients become drowsy and cause circulatory collapse. These drugs are occasionally used sparingly in the critical care unit context, when mechanical ventilation is available. Anxiety is certainly a significant element in many of these cases.

Referral to a critical care unit is appropriate in the above situation. This patient would be at risk from respiratory arrest, and may well need positive pressure ventilation.

The effects of steroids in acute asthma are not immediate. They may not be seen for 6 hours or more after initial administration. It is mandatory to give bronchodilators during this period.

Severe asthma in adults:

Cannot complete sentences
Pulse >110 beats/min
Respiration >25 breaths/min
Peak flow <50% of predicted or best
Consider hospital admission if more than one of the above features is present

Life-threatening asthma:

Silent chest
Cyanosis
Bradycardia or exhaustion
Peak flow <33% of predicted or best

Arrange immediate hospital admission. Consider referral to critical care unit if patient does not respond immediately to treatment.

Indications for Mechanical ventilation in asthma:

Increasing fatigue (increasing pCO_2)
Respiratory failure (rising pCO_2, falling pO_2)
Cardiovascular collapse

The British Thoracic Society. The British guidelines on Asthma management. Thorax 1997 52 (suppl): S1–S21

Singer M, Webb A. Respiratory disorders. In: Oxford Handbook of Critical Care, Oxford University Press, Oxford, 1997

Question 46

A. true **B.** true **C.** true **D.** true **E.** false

The answers to these questions are mostly in Paper 3 Question 45. During the periods of disturbed sleep and apnoeic episodes, hypoxaemia and hypercapnia occur, but not while awake.

Question 47

A. true **B.** true **C.** true **D.** true **E.** false

Contraindications to thoracotomy in lung cancer:

Small cell histology on biopsy or sputum cytology

Evidence of local extrapulmonary invasion:

Hoarseness or bovine cough of laryngeal nerve palsy
Superior vena cava obstruction
Horner's syndrome
Pleural effusion; positive cytology or recurrently blood-stained.

Evidence of mediastinal involvement:

Carinal widening on chest x-ray
Tumour <2cm from carina on bronchoscopy
Positive node biopsy on mediastinoscopy

Evidence of distal spread:

Metastases on liver, bone or brain scan
Malignant cells in bone marrow or CSF

Inability to tolerate surgery

FEV1 <1.2
Pa CO_2 > 45mmHg
Pulmonary Hypertension
Advanced Age

Only about 20% of patients are found to be suitable for surgery on initial assessment and of these only a minority prove respectable. Paraneoplastic syndromes are not contraindications to surgery, and left lung collapse is not evidence of extrapulmonary invasion or mediastinal involvement. The patients are all carefully staged, and all patients with stage IIIb disease are rejected for thoracotomy. Once selected patients have a 5 year survival rate of 30–40%.

Spiro SG. Lung cancer. In Weatherall DJ, Ledingham JGG, Warrell DA, eds. Oxford Textbook of Medicine, Oxford: Oxford University Press, 1996.

Epstein RJ. Medicine for examinations. 3rd Ed. Churchill Livingstone, London, 1996.

Question 48

A. false **B.** true **C.** true **D.** false **E.** true

Helicobacter pylori is a micro-aerophilic, Gram-negative, slow growing, spiral-shaped organism with 4–6 flagellae at one end. H. pylori is probably the most common chronic bacterial infection of humans, present in almost half of the world population, and is usually asymptomatic. Most laboratories in the UK can perform serology and this is an easy bedside test to confirm current or previous infection. Once H. pylori has been eradicated it takes several months (up to 18–20) for antigen levels to decrease, and this is extremely variable. Hence serology is not an ideal measure of response to treatment. The CLO (Campylobacter-Like Organism) test relies on the urease-producing qualities of the organism following biopsy of the gastric mucosa at endoscopy, and is highly sensitive but by definition is invasive. The urea breath test is by far the best non-invasive investigation and is available in some nuclear medicine or gastroenterology units but it is expensive. It relies on detecting urea on the exhaled breath of infected individuals and is highly sensitive. The likely scenario for investigation of H. pylori is the following:

1. The patient has an endoscopy indicated for example by abdominal pain / GI bleed

2. Finding: gastric or duodenal ulcer
3. H. pylori diagnosed at endoscopy by CLO test (or serology if CLO was unavailable)

   If serology is taken in this context it is likely to be useful if the patient has not already had treatment for H. pylori at any stage
4. Eradication of H. pylori by antibiotic triple therapy regimen: PPI e.g. lansoprazole; amoxycillin, and clarithromycin
5. In the context of a GI bleed it is imperative to check for eradication – serology is useless in this context and therefore a urea breath test is preferred.

Although not generally thought of as a nosocomial (hospital acquired) infection there is increasing evidence that all hospital staff, particularly gastroenterologists and endoscopy staff have an increased incidence of infection. The presence of the bacterium in the gastric mucosa is associated with chronic active gastritis and is implicated in more severe gastric diseases, including chronic atrophic gastritis (a precursor of gastric carcinomas), peptic ulceration and mucosa-associated lymphoid tissue lymphomas. Disease outcome depends on many factors, including bacterial genotype, host physiology, genotype and dietary habits.

Robertson MS. Cade JF. Clancy RL. Helicobacter pylori infection in intensive care: increased prevalence and a new nosocomial infection. Critical Care Medicine 1999 27(7): 1276–1280.

Question 49

A. false **B.** true **C.** false **D.** true **E.** false

Small-intestinal lymphangiectasia is rarely seen in adult gastroenterology clinics. The commonest presentation is in children from the primary form, although it presents in adults as secondary to other disease processes such as constrictive pericarditis. Children usually present within the first 2 years with failure to thrive, malabsorption and oedema secondary to low protein.

Essentially it is an immunodeficiency resulting from increased loss of immunoglobulins and lymphocytes from the bowel, the basic defect being an abnormal dilatation of the lymphatic vessels. The hypoproteinaemia is due to abnormal protein loss into the gut.

Clinically there is lymphopenia in the presence of a normal bone marrow and reduction of serum albumin, serum IgG, and carrier proteins such as protein-bound iodine. The protein loss may be accompanied by enteric calcium loss, leading to hypocalcaemia. Steatorrhoea may or may not be present.

Diagnosis depends on showing dilated lymphatics on small bowel biopsy, but the lesion may be patchy and one negative biopsy does not exclude the diagnosis.

Treatment is aimed at reducing long chain fatty acids in the diet leading to a fall in the volume of intestinal lymph and in the pressure of the dilated lymphatics. Occasionally children are unresponsive to this and if the abnormality is extensive throughout the small bowel they may die. Albumin is unhelpful due to its short half-life. Steroids are not used.

Wright VM, Walker-Smith JA. Congenital abnormalities of the gastrointestinal tract. In Weatherall DJ, Ledingham JGG, Warrell DA, eds. Oxford Textbook of Medicine, Oxford: Oxford University Press, 1996.

Question 50

A. true **B.** false **C.** true **D.** false **E.** true

Aphthous ulcers are common with active Crohn's disease, although true oropharyngeal Crohn's ulcers are quite rare. Enteropathic synovitis occurs in 10–20% of patients with Crohn's disease, and patients with HLA B27 tend to have a more axial disease. Ankylosing spondylitis is not characteristic of the disease. Sacroilitis has an increased frequency in Crohn's disease. Primary sclerosing cholangitis is generally associated with ulcerative colitis, however an association has been suggested with Crohn's colitis but the evidence for this has never stood up to close scrutiny. Delayed puberty is common in youngsters with Crohn's.

Extraintestinal manifestations in inflammatory bowel disease

Related to activity of	***Crohn's disease (%)***	***Ulcerative colitis (%)***
Aphthous ulceration	20	less but common
Erythema nodosum	5–10	2
Pyoderma gangrenosum	0.5	1–2
Acute arthropathy	6–12	10–15
Eye complications	3–10	5–8
Conjunctivitis		
Episcleritis		
Uveitis		

Unrelated to disease activity	*Crohn's disease (%)*	*Ulcerative colitis (%)*
Sacroiliitis	15–18	
Ankylosing spondylitis	2–6	
Liver disease		
Sclerosing cholangitis	?exists in CD	3
Gallstones	common	
Chronic active hepatitis	2–3	
Cirrhosis	2–3	
Fatty change	6	60
Cholangiocarcinoma	No	associated
Amyloid, granulomas	rare	even less frequent in UC
Bronchiectasis	No	rare

Epstein RJ. Medicine for examinations. 3rd Ed. Churchill Livingstone, London, 1996.

Question 51

A. true **B.** false **C.** true **D.** false **E.** false

Primary biliary cirrhosis (PBC) is a chronic homeostatic inflammatory liver disease that most commonly affects middle-aged women (90% of PBC patients; generally aged 40–60 years.). It is likely that this is an autoimmune disorder with the discovery of antibodies against mitochondria and in some cases nuclear factors. PBC often has an insidious onset and the diagnosis may only be made after routing blood tests show liver impairment. Classical descriptions of patients with advanced PBC emphasize the presence of clinical cholestasis, with jaundice, pruritus, light stools, easy bruising, and weight loss. Whilst the disease is slow many patients develop cirrhosis and in Europe it is the most common indication for transplantation. 5-year survival following transplant is at least 75% and is constantly improving

Investigations in PBC:

HLA status: there is an association with HLA-DR8.
Elevated ALP (5–20 times normal)
Elevated gamma-GT (if there is any doubt about the ALP being of hepatic origin this lends more weight but of itself it is a non specific test)
Antimitochondrial (M2) antibodies present in 98%. These are highly specific to PBC although M4 antimitochondrial antibodies may occur in autoimmune CAH.
Elevated serum IgM
Elevated cholesterol
Liver biopsy demonstrates chronic inflammation around the bile ducts with granulomas and cirrhosis.
Elevated hepatic copper content

Piecemeal necrosis is characteristic of chronic active hepatitis due for example to hepatitis B (D) and C but also in some cases due to autoimmune CAH or certain drugs.

Prince ME, Jones DE. Primary Biliary Cirrhosis: new perspectives in diagnosis and treatment. Postgraduate Medical Journal 2000 76(894): 199–206

Question 52

A. true **B.** true **C.** true **D.** true **E.** false

Psoriasis is a common, chronic inflammatory skin condition which is relapsing and remitting in nature. Around 2% of the population are affected. It can occur at any age but the mean age of onset is 28. The typical lesion is the formation of a red plaque which in hairy areas has a silvery scale. Psoriasis may be guttate, geographic or circinate. The extensor skin of the elbows and knees are often affected. It can cause palmar plantar pustulosis in which sterile pustules appear on the hands and feet. It exhibits the Koebner phenomenon.

Psoriasis is associated with

- seronegative arthropathy in 5–10%
- nail pitting
- corneal nodules

Trigger factors include

- stress
- trauma
- infection
- lithium
- beta-blockers
- chloroquine

Treatment includes removing the trigger. Topical steroids and coal tar preparations are used. Other treatments are dithranol and PUVA. PUVA consists of UVA light following systemic psoralen. It is associated with an increased risk of skin cancer. Methotrexate is used in very severe cases.

Other causes of the Koebner phenomenon are

- lichen planus
- eczema
- keloid
- sarcoidosis
- viral warts
- vitiligo
- molluscum contagiosum

Berth-Jones J. Psoriasis
Medicine 2000 28; 12: 50–55

Question 53

A. false **B.** false **C.** true **D.** false **E.** true

Klinefelter's syndrome is a developmental disorder of the testis resulting from the presence of an extra X chromosome. The most common karyotype is 47 XXY but rarer variants include 46XY/47 XXY mosaic, multiple X + Y, and the so-called XX male syndrome. The degree of Leydig cell defect is very variable, ranging from the fully virilized male presenting with infertility to the eunuchoidal youth who fails to complete sexual maturation. Gynaecomastia, tall stature, learning difficulties and autoimmune endocrinopathies are features, but not unsteady gait. There is an association with testicular germ-cell tumours.

Causes of gynaecomastia:

Paraneoplastic beta-HCG production
- testicular germ-cell tumour, choriocarcinoma
- adrenal tumours

Primary or secondary hypogonadism

Androgen insensitivity syndromes

Systemic disease
- disseminated malignancy
- malnutrition
- chronic liver disease
- thyrotoxicosis
- renal failure +/– haemodialysis
- leprosy (due to testicular atrophy)
- meningoencephalitic trypanosomiasis
- Wilsons disease

Drugs (normal prolactin)
alcohol (+/– chronic liver disease) due to lowering of plasma testosterone concentrations through a direct toxic effect on Leydig cell steroidogenesis.
oestrogens
antiandrogens
- cyproterone acetate
- spironolactone
- cimetidine

weak oestrogens
- digitoxin
- ketoconazole

Drugs (+/– galactorrhoea, raised prolactin)
methyldopa, reserpine
diamorphine, morphine, marijuana
tricyclics, haloperidol, phenothiazines

Epstein RJ. Medicine for examinations 3rd Ed. London: Churchill Livingstone, 1996.

Question 54

A. false **B.** true **C.** true **D.** false **E.** true

Lipoatrophy is the loss of fat at sites of insulin injection. It is much less common now than in the past when up to 75% of patients treated with insulin were likely to show signs of it. It is said to be due to immunogenic components of conventional insulin preparations that lead to the formation of either immune complexes or IgE antibody, which binds locally and so stimulates lipolysis. It is rare in patients who use highly purified insulins, suggesting that the impurities in older preparations may have contributed to the condition. It tends to happen later in the course of the disease.

Blurred vision may be a symptom of both hyperglycaemia and hypoglycaemia, both of which may result from poor diabetic control, which may occur in the first week of treatment. Hypoglycaemia may cause adrenergic or neuroglycopenic symptoms.

Adrenergic symptoms:
Usually predominate in hypoglycaemia, particularly when the plasma glucose falls rapidly. Adrenaline and other counter-regulatory hormones are secreted and induce pallor, sweating, tremor and palpitations.

Neuroglycopenic symptoms:
Occur when the brain has insufficient glucose. Lack of glucose may induce poor concentration, mood changes, headaches, slow movements, dysarthria, double vision, tingling around the mouth, transient neurological deficits and eventually fits or coma. Each patient has a characteristic group of symptoms that he or she can recognize, and the features may resemble ethanol intoxication.

Pitting oedema may develop within 3 to 4 days of the start of insulin therapy but usually resolves spontaneously 5 to 10 days later. The condition may be severe enough to cause pulmonary oedema.

Although the cause is unknown, sodium retention may occur, and plasma albumin is generally normal. Insulin oedema is not common, but is extremely troublesome. It is seen when proper glycaemic control is achieved in markedly hyperglycaemic and underweight diabetics.

Insulin allergy is either local or general and is rare. The local form causes pruritic, erythematous indurated and occasionally painful lesions after insulin injection. The incidence is decreased in those using highly purified insulins. Generalized allergy is extremely rare and presents as a classical anaphylactic reaction. A photosensitivity rash is not a feature of insulin allergy.

Bell JI, Hockaday TDR. Diabetes Mellitus. In Weatherall DJ, Ledingham JGG, Warrell DA, eds. Oxford Textbook of Medicine, Oxford: Oxford University Press, 1996.

Question 55

A. true **B.** false **C.** true **D.** true **E.** false

See Paper 2 Question 53 for further discussion on polycystic ovary syndrome.

Question 56

A. true **B.** true **C.** false **D.** true **E.** true

Ocular involvement is one of the hallmarks of the clinical syndrome of Graves' disease. The proptosis (abnormal protrusion of the eyeball, caused by enlarging retro-orbital tissue), ophthalmoplegia, chemosis (collection of fluid under the conjunctiva covering the white of the eye so it balloons forward) and increased retro-orbital pressure can lead to papilloedema, optic atrophy or loss of vision (described as malignant exophthalmos).

The condition is usually bilateral, although is often asymmetrical and may be unilateral; in this case it may be confused with a retro-orbital tumour. The eye signs may occur in the absence of overt hyperthyroidism or even after its successful treatment. The cause of the ophthalmopathic form of hyperthyroidism is not understood. Excess secretion of TSH is not responsible. Pathologically there is retro-orbital deposition of mucopolysaccharides with oedema and round-cell infiltration, thickened extra-ocular muscles may be demonstrated on CT scan.

Xerophthalmia is dryness of the eyes with thickening of the conjunctiva occurring in vitamin A deficiency, pemphigus and autoimmune disorders such as Sjogren's syndrome. Artificial tears must be used constantly to maintain the essential film of water over the cornea.

Wartofsky L. Diseases of the Thyroid. In Isselbacher KJ, Braunwald E, Wilson JD et al., eds. Harrisons Principles of Internal Medicine, 13th Edition. New York: McGraw-Hill, 1994.

Weetman AP. Grave's disease
NEJM 2000 343: 17; 1236–1248

Question 57

A. false **B.** false **C.** true **D.** true **E.** false

This question relies on being able to calculate the anion gap and knowing the causes of a raised or normal anion gap acidosis. The anion gap is the sum of (Na + K) – (Cl + HCO3) and is normally between 10–18. In this question the anion gap is raised at 28.1

Causes of a raised anion gap acidosis include:

lactic acidosis
diabetic ketoacidosis
acute or chronic renal failure
hepatic failure
salicylate poisoning
methanol or ethylene glycol ingestion

Causes of a normal anion gap acidosis include:

renal tubular acidosis
severe diarrhoea
high-output fistulae
utero sigmoidostomy
acetazolamide
hypoaldosteronism.

Bartter's syndrome is a rare metabolic disorder that results in hyperaldosteronism without hypertension. Typical findings are hyperaldosteronism, hypereninaemia, and hypokalaemic metabolic alkalosis. Treatment is supportive with potassium supplementation, potassium sparing diuretics, and in severe cases prostaglandin synthetase inhibitors such as Indomethacin.

Forrest DM, Russell JA. Metabolic Acidosis.
Webb RA et al. Oxford Textbook of Critical Care. 1999 Oxford University Press. Oxford.

Question 58

A. false **B.** false **C.** true **D.** true **E.** false

Adult polycystic kidney disease is a common disorder accounting for up to 10% of cases of endstage renal failure. 90% of cases are inherited in an autosomal dominant manner with the other 10% occurring sporadically. The kidneys are grossly enlarged with multiple cysts of varying size distributed throughout the cortex and medulla. Hepatic cysts occur in up to 75% of cases and berry aneurysms in 10%. There is also an increased incidence of colonic diverticular disease, mitral valve prolapse and aortic regurgitation.

The disease may present with acute abdominal pain due to haemorrhage into a cyst, chronic flank discomfort, abdominal mass, haematuria, nephrolithiasis, hypertension (present in 75% of cases), or recurrent urinary tract infections. 50% of patients develop endstage renal failure by the age of 60.

The diagnosis is usually by ultrasound scanning with the diagnostic criteria being the presence of at least 3–5 cysts in each kidney. Ultrasound scanning is also used to identify familial cases with genetic linkage analysis (gene locus short arm of chromosome 16) reserved for screening family members with a negative scan if a definite diagnosis is required eg. prior to kidney donation.

Grunfeld JP Clinical aspects of inherited renal disorders.

Ledingham JGG, Warrell DA. Concise Oxford Textbook of Clinical Medicine. 2000. Oxford University Press. Oxford.

Question 59

A. false **B.** true **C.** true **D.** false **E.** false

Acute nephritic syndrome comprises haematuria, proteinuria, oliguria, oedema, and hypertension. It is the clinical picture that develops in response to an acute glomerulonephritis. Thus it can occur either in response to a primary glomerulonephritis or as part of a more generalized vasculitis. Membranous and minimal change glomerulonephritis present with the nephrotic syndrome and not nephritis.

Causes of the nephritic syndrome –

Diffuse Proliferative glomerulonephritis: idiopathic, post-streptococcal glomerulonephritis

Focal segmental glomerulonephritis: primary renal disease or secondary to SBE, shunt nephritis, SLE, Henoch-Schonlein purpura, IgA nephropathy, microscopic polyarteritis, Wegener's granulomatosis

Proliferative glomerulonephritis with crescent formation: Goodpasture's syndrome, Wegener's granulomatosis, microscopic polyarteritis

Mesangiocapillary nephritis: idiopathic, shunt nephritis, partial lipodystrophy

Alport's syndrome

Cameron JS. Common Clinical Presentations and Symptoms in Renal Disorders
Ledingham JGG, Warrell DA (Eds). Concise Oxford textbook of Medicine. 2000 Oxford University Press, Oxford

Question 60

A. true **B.** true **C.** false **D.** true **E.** true

This question simply requires linking the given information with causes of chronic renal failure.

Childhood haematuria could be related to glomerulonephritis or recurrent urinary tract infections and the development of reflux nephropathy. Berry aneurysms are associated with adult polycystic kidney disease. NSAIDS can cause acute and chronic interstitial nephritis (analgesic nephropathy). Bronchiectasis predispose patients to the development of reactive AA amyloidosis and the development of renal failure.

Haemolytic disease of the newborn is due to maternal red cell antibodies passing into the fetal circulation and destroying fetal red cells. ABO or RhD incompatibility are the commonest causes. There is no association with renal failure.

Nahas AMEl, Winearls CG. Chronic Renal Failure
Oxford Textbook of Medicine. Oxford University Press.

Paper 6 Answers

Question 1

A. true **B.** true **C.** true **D.** true **E.** true

Homocystinuria is characterised by an increase in homocysteine and homocystine, which accumulate proximal to the metabolic block, caused by a deficiency in the enzyme cystathionine beta synthase. The gene encoding this enzyme resides on chromosome 21; the condition is inherited as autosomal recessive. Homocystinuria is an important differential diagnosis for Marfans – a condition for which it shares many phenotypic features. Features include:

Ocular	downward dislocation of the lens myopia glaucoma retinal degeneration and detachment cataracts optic atrophy corneal abnormalities
Skeletal	similar to Marfan's syndrome long thin habitus pectus excavatum scoliosis and genu valgum osteoporosis / spontaneous vertebral crush fractures
CNS	reduced IQ seizures strokes

The common abnormalities seen in Marfan's syndrome – high arched palate, pectus excavatum or carinatum, genu valgum, pes cavus or planus, scoliosis – are all well recognized in homocystinuria. Arachnodactyly is less common and the fingers not infrequently (and elbows occasionally) show mild flexion contractures. Skeletal disproportion with a crown pubis length less than the pubis heel length is usual. Diagnosis is by the cyanide nitroprusside test performed on urine. Treatment consists of: a) pyridoxine (vitamin B6) in those who respond to pyridoxine and b) methionine restriction in those who do not respond to pyridoxine.

Major risk factors for venous thrombosis, particularly of the lower limbs and pelvis:

recent surgery/tissue trauma
immobility for more than 3 or 4 days
age over 40 years
previous venous thrombosis and / or embolism
presence or suspicion of malignant disease
sepsis
obesity
varicose veins

The risk of venous thrombosis, and therefore of resultant pulmonary embolism is increased in:

pregnancy
the puerperium
young women taking the oral contraceptive pill
the nephrotic syndrome.

Rare conditions that increase the risk of venous disease include:

paroxysmal nocturnal haemoglobinuria
homocystinuria
Behçet's disease
lupus anticoagulant
deficiency of antithrombin III, proteins C or S
resistance to activated protein C

Differences between Marfan's and Homocystinuria

Phenotype	**Marfans**	**Homocystinuria**
inheritance	AD	AR
osteoporosis	no	yes
skeletal disproportion	no	yes
thrombotic tendency	no	yes
platelet adhesion disorder	yes	no
lens dislocation	upward	downwards
chromosome defect	15	21
IQ	normal	reduced in some cases
neurological abnormalities	no	yes
arachnodactyly	yes	less common
colonic diverticulae	yes	no
dissection of the aorta	yes	no
mitral valve prolapse	yes	no
parenchymal lung disease	yes	no
main cause of death	cardiovascular	thrombotic

See Paper 4 Question 2 for a discussion on Marfan's syndrome.

Smith R. Disorders of the skeleton
Oxford Textbook of Medicine. Oxford University Press.

Question 2

A. true **B.** false **C.** false **D.** true **E.** false

X linked recessive disorders:

Agammaglobulinaemia
Anhidrotic ectodermal dysplasia
Becker muscular dystrophy
Colour blindness
Duchenne muscular dystrophy
Fabry's disease
G-6-PD deficiency
Haemophilia A & B
Hunter's syndrome
Lesch-Nyhan disease
Menkes syndrome
Mental retardation
Ocular albinism

Wiskott Aldrich syndrome

Dominant X linked:

Incontinentia pigmenti
Orofacial-digital syndrome
Vitamin D-resistant rickets

Kingston HM. ABC of Clinical genetics
British Medical Journal Publishing

Pembrey ME. Genetic factors in disease
Oxford Textbook of Medicine. Oxford University Press

Question 3

A. true **B.** true **C.** false **D.** false **E.** true

Olfactory nerve. Any frontal lobe tumours e.g. olfactory groove meningiomas may lead to unilateral anosmia secondary to direct compression of the nerve. Bilateral anosmia or impairment is common with the common cold or sinusitis; head injuries affecting the cribriform plate and heavy smokers.

Vestibular nerve. Any unilateral lesion e.g. occlusion of blood supply, acoustic neuroma etc of the cochlear nucleus of the VIIIth nerve will produce unilateral deafness.

Facial nerve. Sparing of the frontalis muscle will occur in an upper motor neurone lesion.

Eye muscles lesions

Direction of weakness	Nerve Supply
up and out	III
up and in	III
medially	III
down and out	III
down and in	IV
laterally	VI

The third cranial nerve supplies all the muscles of the eye except the superior oblique (IVth) and lateral rectus (VIth). From the midbrain it enters the orbit through the common tendinous ring and divides into an upper division for the superior rectus and the levator palpebrae superioris and a lower division for the medial and inferior rectus and the inferior oblique. The latter branch carries an important parasympathetic contribution to the ciliary ganglion, which after synapsing, supplies the sphincter pupillae (constriction of the pupil) and the ciliary muscle of the eye, the muscle of accommodation or focus. These autonomic fibres come from the Edinger Westphal nucleus of the midbrain.

Clinically a complete IIIrd nerve palsy manifests as:

1. ptosis
2. after lifting the eyelid there is divergent strabismus and a dilated pupil. The eye is fixed in a down and out position.

Causes of a complete IIIrd nerve palsy:

unruptured aneurysm of posterior communicating artery
mononeuritis multiplex
midbrain vascular lesion
mibrain demylinating lesion
meningovascular syphilis
opthalmoplegic migraine
encephalitis
parasellar neoplasms
sphenoidal wing meningiomas
carcinomatous lesions of the skull base

Causes of mononeuritis multiplex:

diabetes mellitus
polyarteritis nodosa
Churg-Strauss syndrome
rheumatoid arthritis
SLE
Wegener's granulomatosis
sarcoidosis
carcinoma
amyloidosis

Scadding JW, Gibby J. Neurological disease
Oxford Textbook of Medicine. Oxford University Press.

Question 4

A. true **B.** false **C.** true **D.** false **E.** false

Abductor pollicis is supplied by the ulnar nerve. The fist dorsal interosseous is supplied by the median nerve. Convention in anatomical teaching dictates that the naming of the fingers of the hand are best done in individual terms rather than numerically (e.g. thumb (1st), Index (2nd) Middle (3rd) Ring (4th) and little finger (5th). Sensation of the 1st, 2nd, and 3rd digits is therefore the median, the ulnar supplies the 5th (little) finger and medial aspect of the 4th (ring) finger. Clinical examples of nerve lesions:

Median (cut at the wrist): loss of sensation of all the thenar and distal aspects of the lateral three and a half fingers, loss of opposition of the thumb, weakness of two lumbricals (but this is compensated for by the interossei)

Ulnar (at the wrist): loss of the hypothenar muscles, 1st two ulnar lumbricals, loss of all the interossei with the inability to oppose and separate the fingers, loss of sensation to the medial one and a half fingers

Ulnar (at the elbow): palpable thickening of the nerve in the ulnar groove, sparing of muscles of the forearm, wasting of the first dorsal interosseous and abductor digiti minimi, wasting of the other interossei, claw hand posture

Scadding JW, Gibby J. Neurological disease
Oxford Textbook of Medicine. Oxford University Press.

Question 5

A. true **B.** true **C.** true **D.** true **E.** true

Relationship between hypothalamic and pituitary hormones:

Hypothalamic	***pituitary hormone***	***Target gland***	***Feedback***
TRH	TSH	thyroid gland	T4/T3
GnRH	LH/FSH	gonads	oestradiol & testosterone
SS	GH	multiple	IGF-1
DA	PRL	breast	
CRH	ACTH	adrenal	cortisol
AVP	ACTH	adrenal	cortisol
GHRH	GH	multiple	IGF-1

TRH	thyrotrophin releasing hormone
TSH	thyroid stimulating hormone

T4	thyroxine
T3	tri-iodothyronine
GnRH	gonadotrophin releasing hormone
FSH	follicle stimulating hormone
LH	leuteinizing hormone
SS	hypothalamic somatostatin
GH	growth hormone
IGF-1	insulin growth factor I
DA	hypothalamic dopamine
PRL	prolactin
CRH	corticotrophin releasing hormone
ACTH	adrenocorticotrophin
AVP	vasopressin
GHRH	growth hormone releasing hormone

Each pituitary hormone is regulated by substances which are synthesized in the hypothalamus and transported from the median eminence to the anterior pituitary via the hypothalamic – pituitary portal circulation. Each of these hypothalamic regulatory hormones bind to specific high affinity cell membrane receptors of the particular pituitary cell type to regulate pituitary hormone secretion. All of the anterior pituitary hormones are also regulated (by negative feedback) by the hormones secreted by their target glands.

Roles of the hypothalamus

1. temperature regulation
   IL-1, TNF-alpha, IL-6 all induce prostaglandin synthesis in the hypothalamus; all are pyogenic
2. appetite
3. fluid and electrolyte balance: the hypothalamus contains osmoreceptors and also manufactures vasopressin which is released in the posterior hyothalamus
4. completion of feedback loops e.g. with oestrogen and progesterone feeding back in the hypothalamus / pituitary the menstrual cycle is created
5. thirst

Thorner MO. Anterior Pituitary Disorders
Oxford Textbook of Medicine. Oxford University Press.

Question 6

A. false **B.** true **C.** false **D.** true **E.** false

Prostacyclin (PGI-2) actions:

1. potent vasodilator (secreted by endothelium) liberated by shear stress applied to endothelial cells
2. antiaggregator – potent inhibitor of platelet aggregation, adhesion and secretion
3. natriuretic

Mackie IJ. The biology of haemostasis and thrombosis
Oxford Textbook of Medicine. Oxford University Press.

Question 7

A. false **B.** false **C.** true **D.** true **E.** false

Short term metabolic effects of some hormones:

Insulin	increases glucose transport (not liver) glycogen synthesis protein synthesis lipogenesis esterification decreases lipolysis gluconeogenesis
Glucagon	increases glycogen breakdown gluconeogenesis alanine transport (liver) lipolysis ketogenesis decreases esterification lipogenesis
Catecholamines	increases glycogen breakdown gluconeogenesis glycolysis lipolysis ketogenesis decreases esterification

Insulin acts to lower glucose, fatty acids, ketone bodies and amino acids. Glucagon and catecholamines serve to increase glucose, fatty acids and ketone bodies and, in the case of catecholamines, lactate.

Smith R, Williamsone DH. Biochemical background.
Oxford Textbook of Medicine. Oxford University Press.

Question 8

A. false **B.** false **C.** false **D.** true **E.** false

See Paper 3 Questions 7 & 8.

Renin is secreted by the juxta-glomerular apparatus in the kidney; it converts angiotensinogen (manufactured in the liver) to angiotensin I. Angiotensin I is converted to angiotensin II by the angiotensin converting enzyme (ACE) found in peripheral tissues and in the lung. Angiotensin II in addition to the extracellular salt and potassium concentration stimulates the release of aldosterone.

Causes of hypokalaemia:

Intracellular shifts:	alkalosis high dose insulin beta-2 adrenergic stimulation toluene intoxication (glue sniffing)
Renal wasting	metabolic and respiratory alkalosis diuretics solute diuresis e.g. mannitol aldosteronism: primary / secondary / renin secreting tumours Cushing's syndrome adrenogenital syndromes Bartter's syndrome Liddle's syndrome magnesium depletion carbenoxolone liquorice addiction renal tubular acidosis ureterosigmoidostomy genatamicin amikacin acute leukaemia
Gastrointestinal	pyloric stenosis bulimia / anorexia nervosa ileostomy chloride diarrhoea villous adenoma of rectum purgative abuse

Ledingham JGG. Disorders of potassium metabolism Oxford Textbook of Medicine. Oxford University Press.

Question 9

A. true **B.** true **C.** true **D.** false **E.** true

Summary of events during inspiration:

1. decreased intrathoracic pressure (negative pressure)
2. increased blood flow in SVC / IVC to the right atria and right ventricle towards lungs (hence prolongation of right ventricular systole)
3. decreased blood flow to left side of heart and hence to the aorta
4. accentuation of right sided murmurs
5. diminution of left sided murmurs
6. fall in jugular venous pressure

Pride NB. Lung fuction testing
Oxford Textbook of Medicine. Oxford University Press.

Question 10

A. true **B.** false **C.** true **D.** false **E.** true

Causes of a metabolic acidosis with a normal anion gap:

renal tubular acidosis	
gastrointestinal causes:	diarrhoea pancreatic/biliary fistula
ureteroenterostomy	+/– obstructed ileal bladder & vesico-iliocolic fistula
iatrogenic	acetazolamide cholestryamine parenteral

Causes of a metabolic acidosis and a normal anion gap with hyperkalaemia:

Type IV renal tubular acidosis
treated diabetic ketoacidosis
obstructive uropathy
early uraemic acidosis
mineralocorticoid deficiency

Causes of a high anion gap:

uraemia

predominant ketoacidosis (diabetic / alcoholic / starvation)

predominant type A lactic acidosis	e.g. exercise post epileptic shock-trauma, haemorrhagic, cardiogenic, septic hypoxia (severe)
predominant type B lactic acidosis	biguanides severe liver disease paracetamol poisoning thiamine deficiency
overdose	e.g. with aspirin (acidotic phase) methanol ethylene glycol paraldehyde Reye's syndrome

To calculate the anion gap you need to measure the following: plasma sodium, potassium, chloride, (from a standard U & E screen) and bicarbonate (usually from blood gases). Use of the anion gap: the sum of the measured cations (Na^+ and K^+) normally exceeds that of the measured anions (Cl^- and HCO_3^-) by about 14mmol/litre (reference range 10 to 18mmol/l).

$[Na + K] > [Cl + HCO_3]$ by14

This difference is known as the anion gap; and is attributable largely to negatively charged proteins but also to phosphate, sulphate, and some organic acids. Calculation of the anion gap is principally of value in the differential diagnosis of metabolic acidosis and in following the progress of therapy. Metabolic acidosis may be divided broadly into those with normal and those with high anion gap.

Metabolic acidosis with normal anion gap: these are due to the direct loss of bicarbonate from the body, either through the gut (e.g. diarrhoea, pancreatic fistulae, ureterosigmoidostomy) or through the kidney (e.g. renal tubular acidosis, acetazolamide therapy) or, rarely to the ingestion or infusion of hydrochloric acid or substances effectively giving rise to it (e.g. ammonium chloride, arginine hydrochloride). When bicarbonate is lost more chloride is retained by the renal tubules; thus low plasma bicarbonate is accompanied by hyperchloraemia and the anion gap remains unaltered. In the case of hydrochloric acid intake bicarbonate is titrated and replaced by chloride.

Metabolic acidosis with high anion gap: these are due to the ingestion or endogenous generation of organic acids, whose anions are not routinely measured. Plasma bicarbonate is titrated and the anion gap is now widened by the presence of these unmeasured anions. The principal causes are ketoacidosis, lactic acidosis, uraemic acidosis, and poisoning by salicylates. In uraemic acidosis the anion gap seldom exceeds 28mmol/l, but considerably higher values may be found in severe lactic acidosis and ketoacidosis. It should be noted that there are causes of raised anion gap other than metabolic acidosis, for example therapy with sodium salts of relatively strong acids (e.g. lactate, acetate) and high-dose sodium carbenicillin therapy, and respiratory or metabolic alkalosis.

Cohen RD, Woods HF. Disturbances of acid-base homeostasis. Oxford Textbook of Medicine. Oxford University Press.

Question 11

A. true **B.** true **C.** false **D.** false **E.** false

Some antibodies and disease associations

Antibody	***Disease Association***
Anti-dsDNA, Anti-Sm, Anti-U1RNP	SLE
Anti-Ro and La	
Anti-Ro and La	Sjogren's
cANCA	Wegener's
pANCA	PAN/UC
thyroid microsomal antibodies	hypothyroidism
streptococcal antibodies	acute rheumatic fever
antibodies to M2 antigen	primary biliary cirrhosis
ANA/SMA autoantibodies	chronic active (autoimmune) hepatitis
anti-endothelial autoantibodies	IDDM, Raynaud's disease systemic sclerosis Kawasaki disease haemolytic uraemic syndrome transplant rejection
Jo-1 antibodies	myositis
antiglomerular basement membrane antibodies	Goodpasture's syndrome
antineutrophil cytoplasmic antibodies	systemic vasculitis
antiparietal cell, intrinsic factor antibodies	B12
warm/cold antibodies	autoimmune haemolytic anaemia
antiphospholipid antibodies	acute self limiting infections syphilis malaria HIV infection Hepatitis C infection SLE / systemic sclerosis rheumatoid arthritis temporal arthritis psoriatic arthropathy

Epstein RJ. Medicine for Examinations
Churchill Livingstone 1996 London

Question 12

A. false **B.** true **C.** true **D.** false **E.** false

Patients with common varied immunodeficiency (CVID) or common variable hypogammaglobulinaemia present at any age, with a peak incidence in early childhood and in late adolescence. Serum immunoglobulin levels are variable, but usually serum IgA is virtually absent, and the IgG and IgM are both low. Occasionally some have a normal or raised IgM levels. Relatives of the index case may also be affected with an increased incidence of selective IgA deficiency and/or autoimmune disease in first-degree relatives, and occasionally a parent and offspring may both develop CVID. In around 50% of cases the C4A*QO, DR3; the same haplotype is associated with systemic lupus erythematosus, coeliac disease, and a poor prognosis in human immunodeficiency virus (HIV) infection. One third of patients have a profound depletion of lymphocytes with low CD4+ T-cell counts and B cells, and a relative increase in CD8 T cells; similar phenotypic changes are seen in AIDS. This subgroup tend to have splenomegaly and sometimes hypersplenism, and a few have recurrent lymphadenopathy. Despite all the low counts documented above the prognosis is relatively good and only about 10 per cent die from opportunistic fungal and viral infections within 30 years from onset of symptoms. Patients with CVID are prone to mycoplasmas and certain bacterial, protozoal, and viral infections.

Classification of some primary immunodeficiencies:

ANTIBODY DEFICIENCY
X-linked agammaglobulinaemia
Common varied immunodeficiency
Thymoma with hypogammaglobulinaemia
Selective IgA deficiency
Selective IgG subclass deficiencies
Transient hypogammaglobulinaemia of infancy

SELECTIVE T-CELL DEFICIENCY
Thymic aplasia
Purine nucleoside phosphorylase deficiency
T-cell-receptor defects

MIXED T- AND B-CELL DEFECTS
Severe: Severe combined immunodeficiency:
X-linked
adenosine deaminase deficiency
lymphocyte class II deficiency

Moderate Immunodeficiency with hyper-IgM
Ataxia telangiectasia
Wiskott-Aldrich disease

Webster ADB. Immunodeficiency
Oxford Textbook of Medicine. Oxford University Press.

Question 13

A. false **B.** true **C.** true **D.** false **E.** true

There are two basic types of immune response:

humoral response: based on B lymphocytes which produce antibodies

cell mediated: dependent on T lymphocytes.

Immune response from antibodies can be silent e.g. neutralizing virus infectivity but occasionally visible at the bed side if they trigger secondary events (e.g. anaphylaxis). Cell mediated immune responses can be silent too (clearing virus infection by T cells lysing infected cells), visible (e.g. by delayed hypersensitivity in the skin) or revealed by investigation (e.g. kidney graft refection). Both B and T cells interact with each other and also with antigen presenting cells. Unlike B cells, T cells will not respond to antigen which is soluble or free but only to antigen at the cell surface. The antigen must be protein derived and linked or associated with histocompatibility molecules (HLA). In the case of the T helper cells the HLA class II will be expressed on antigen presenting cells e.g. macrophages. The role of the antigen presenting macrophages is to capture protein, ingest it, process it internally and present it in this processed form on its surface in association with HLA class II. From a previous question we saw that T lymphocytes can be split basically into T helper cells and cytotoxic T cells. T helper cells (Th cells) recognise HLA class II (and when foreign antigen is presented to them) will stimulate B cells to make antibody. Th1 and Th2 cells secrete a variety of cytokines including interleukins and interferon. The other chief subset of T cells, the cytotoxic T lymphocytes will recognise foreign antigen at the surface of non-specialized presenting cells e.g. a cell infected by a virus. In this case there will be peptide fragments of the virus present on the cell surface in association with HLA class I molecules (not class II) and the cytotoxic T cells recognise the peptide HLA class I complex.

Delves PJ, Roitt IM. The Immune System I & II
NEJM 2000 343: 1; 37–49 & NEJM 2000 343: 2; 108–117

Medzhitov R, Janeway C. Innate immunity
NEJM 2000 343: 5; 338–344

Question 14

A. true **B.** true **C.** true **D.** false **E.** false

Toxoplasma gondii is a protozoan organism that typically infects cats. Ingestion of oocysts excreted by cats or present in the meat of infected livestock leads to the development of toxoplasmosis in man. Ingested cysts release sporozoites in the gut which then spread via the blood stream and lymphatics throughout the body.

Infection is usually subclinical though a febrile illness with lymphadenopathy, mild hepatitis, and splenomegaly mimicking glandular fever can develop. In immunosuppressed subjects a more severe illness usually develops. Infection of the CNS can cause encephalitis, multiple space-occupying lesions in the brain, seizures, and psychiatric disturbance. Infection in-utero can lead to spontaneous abortion or severe congenital toxoplasmosis. The risk of fetal death is highest with infection during the 3rd trimester though conversely the risk of severe congenital infection is highest during the 1st. Features include hydrocephalus, microcephaly, choroidoretinitis, cerebral calcification, and multiorgan involvement.

Choroidoretinitis can occur following congenital or acquired toxoplasmosis. It may simply present as loss of vision in later childhood. Diagnosis is by serology or demonstration of the parasite in infected body tissue. IgM antibody may be present for up to a year following infection so serology based on acute phase IgG antibody is used to distinguish between acute and past infection. Treatment is pyrimethamine and sulphadiazine. These can cause bone marrow depression which may be prevented by the addition of folic acid. Regular blood monitoring is necessary. Pregnant women should receive spiramycin instead of pyrimethamine.

Weller IVD, Conlon CP, Peto TEA. HIV infection and AIDS
Oxford Textbook of Medicine. Oxford University Press.

Question 15

A. false **B.** true **C.** true **D.** false **E.** false

For discussion on infectious mononucleosis see Paper 5 Question 14.

Question 16

A. true **B.** false **C.** false **D.** true **E.** false

Hepatitis C virus is a single stranded RNA virus transmitted directly through needle inoculation or transfusion of contaminated blood products, or indirectly either during intercourse or at birth. Six different genotypes exist with type 1, 2, and 3 accounting for nearly all the cases in Britain. The seroprevalence varies between different population groups and in U.K. ranges from 0.04% in blood donors to 1% in genitourinary clinics. Acute infection is usually sub-clinical with 80% of subjects subsequently becoming chronic carriers. The natural history of chronic infection is unclear though on liver biopsy up to 70% have evidence of chronic active hepatitis with between 15–20% eventually progressing to cirrhosis, and end-stage liver disease. One third of patients however may not progress at all. Liver function tests are not predictive of the degree of liver damage making liver biopsy essential to guiding management. Chronic Hepatitis C infection is a risk factor for the development of hepatocellular carcinoma and in some countries such as Japan it is now the major cause. Diagnosis is by serological testing. Positive ELISA tests should be confirmed by a recombinant immunoblot assay (RIBA) or by HCV PCR to exclude false positive results and subjects who have cleared the virus. Guidelines on treatment in the U.K. have recently been published by NICE (National Institute for Clinical Excellence). Treatment is recommended for patients with moderate to severe Hepatitis C with evidence of inflammation or fibrosis on biopsy. Combination therapy with Ribavirin and Interferon alpha should initially be given for 6 months with a further 6 months for patients with type 1 genotype whose viral RNA is undetectable after the initial treatment. Response rates are nearly twice as high in patients infected with genotypes 2 and 3 compared to genotype 1 with overall an approximately 40% sustained response to treatment at one year. Factors predictive of a sustained response include young age, female sex, genotype 2 or 3, and a lesser degree of fibrosis on liver biopsy.

Side-effects of combination therapy include haemolysis, anaemia, pruritus, cough and depression. Ribavarin is also known to be teratogenic and adequate birth control measures must be taken during treatment and for at least 6 months afterwards.

Liang TJ, Rehermann B, Seeff LB, et al. Pathogenesis, Natural History, Treatment, and Prevention of Hepatitis C. Annals of Internal Medicine. 2000 132(4): 296–305

Question 17

A. true **B.** false **C.** true **D.** false **E.** false

For a discussion on the benign malarias see Paper 4 Question 16.

For a discussion on Plasmodium falciparum see Paper 5 Question 17.

Question 18

A. true **B.** false **C.** true **D.** false **E.** true

See earlier question on factor VIII: Paper 4 Question 19.

Question 19

A. false **B.** false **C.** true **D.** true **E.** false

Folate deficiency is a cause of macrocytic anaemia.

The blood film shows hypersegmented neutrophils.

It causes glossitis

Leucoerythroblastic blood film (presence of red and white cell precursors): variable degree of anaemia, changes in shape and size of the red cells, and the presence of nucleated red cells plus metamyelocytes, myelocytes or even myeloblasts in the peripheral blood. Some causes include:

1. Myelofibrosis
2. Marrow infiltration

For example: metastases (eg commonly seen in breast/prostate)

myeloma
malignant lymphoma
marble bone disease (osteopetrosis)
metabolic: Gauchers disease

Weatherall DJ. Myelosclerosis
Oxford Textbook of Medicine. Oxford University Press.

Question 20

A. false **B.** true **C.** false **D.** false **E.** false

Thrombocytopenia

There is no relation between the speed of recovery and the severity of thrombocytopenia at presentation in patients with ITP. Neonatal alloimmune thrombocytopenia occurs when there is incompatibility between parental and fetal platelet antigens. Maternal antibodies react with neonatal platelets in utero causing fetal thrombocytopenia. It can be severe and life threatening.

Henoch Schönlein purpura is a leukocytoclastic vasculitis. The purpura is not of haematological origin. It usually affects children between 2 and 8 years old. It often presents 1–3 weeks after an upper respiratory tract infection. There is a rapid onset of a palpable purpuric rash over the extensor aspect of the buttocks and legs. It may be associated with abdominal pain. There can be an arthritis particularly affecting the ankles and knees. Renal involvement can occur usually in the form of haematuria and proteinuria. It can progress to chronic renal failure. It usually resolves spontaneously but troublesome joint pains may be treated with steroids.

Uraemia is associated with platelet dysfunction but not a reduction in the platelet count. Aspirin inhibits platelet aggregation not paracetamol.

Epstein RJ. Medicine for examinations
Churchill Livingstone

Question 21

A. false **B.** true **C.** false **D.** false **E.** false

Primary polycythaemia is a stem cell disorder. There is excess proliferation of erythroid, myeloid and megakaryocytic progenitor cells. There is an increase in haemoglobin and PCV, the white cell count is elevated in around 70% of cases and platelets are high in around 50%.

Clinical problems arise due to increased plasma viscosity and volume. The patient is often plethoric and suffers a severe pruritus especially if warm. The mechanism of the latter is unclear but it is not due to bile salt retention. There is an increased incidence of gout due to increase in cell turnover. Thrombosis and haemorrhage are the major complications.

Diagnosis is confirmed by

- Increased Hb and PCV
- Increased megakaryocytes and erythroid hyperplasia on bone marrow
- Increased red cell volume
- Raised Leucocyte alkaline phosphatase (LAP) score
- Increased serum vit B12 and its binding protein hydroxycobalamin

Causes of a raised LAP score include

- Osteomyelofibrosis
- Polycythaemia rubra vera
- Myeloid reactions
- Increased serum vit B12 and its binding protein

Epstein RJ. Medicine for examinations
Churchill Livingstone

Question 22

A. true **B.** true **C.** false **D.** true **E.** true

Major adverse effects recognized with non-steroidal anti-inflammatory drugs (NSAIDs) are

- Gastrointestinal: namely peptic ulceration and erosions
- Prolonged bleeding time: this is due to impaired platelet aggregation and inhibition of the thromboxane system
- Bronchospasm
- Salt retention and an increase in extracellular volume
- Renal failure: papillary necrosis, interstitial fibrosis that can cause nephrotic syndrome
- Pancreatitis
- Worsening of colitis
- Diarrhoea
- Photosensitivity

Amadio P, Cummings DM, Amadio PB. NSAIDs revisited: selection, monitoring, and safe use. Postgraduate Medicine 1997 101(2): 257–271

Question 23

A. true **B.** false **C.** false **D.** false **E.** true

The major drugs causing gingival hypertrophy are

cyclosporin
phenytoin
nifedipine
oral contraceptive

Other conditions causing gingival hypertrophy include

scurvy
heavy metal poisoning
leukaemia
pregnancy

Burton JL, Healey CJ. Aids to Postgraduate Medicine
Sixth Edition, Churchill Livingstone 1994

Question 24

A. true **B.** true **C.** true **D.** true **E.** true

Erythromycin inhibits the metabolism of cisapride leading to an increase in the incidence of arrhythmias. Cisapride is associated with prolongation of the QT interval. Although voluntarily withdrawn from the world market it is still available on a named patient basis.

The co prescribing of gentamicin and frusemide is associated with increased ototoxicity.

Ciprofloxacin is an enzyme inhibitor and as such potentiates the effect of warfarin.

Metronidazole inhibits the metabolism of phenytoin. Phenytoin has a narrow therapeutic index and so combination treatment may cause increased side effects and toxicity.

British National Formulary
Published by BMA and Royal Pharmaceutical Society of Great Britain

Question 25

A. true **B.** false **C.** true **D.** true **E.** true

Impaired renal function influences drug therapy in several ways.

1. May worsen the existing condition
2. May increase the incidence of side effects
3. The effect of the drug may be altered
4. The pharmacokinetics may be changed. There is a decrease in the excretion of renally eliminated drugs. There may be altered protein binding.

With respect to the altered pharmacokinetics the clinician may need to

1. Decrease the dose
2. Alter the dosing interval
3. Prescribe a loading dose to obtain satisfactory levels
4. Perform more frequent monitoring for instance amino glycosides and digoxin

Decreased binding is especially relevant with phenytoin. A different therapeutic range is used in renal impairment.

There may be an altered drug effect. This appears to be independent of the pharmacokinetics. Examples of this include opiates, barbiturates and benzodiazepines. Antihypertensives exert a more postural effect.

Renal failure may be worsened by the administration of nephrotoxic drugs such as ceftazidime. It may also be worsened by drugs causing fluid retention such as NSAIDs. The level of uraemia is increased by some agents such as tetracyclines and corticosteroids. There may be an increase in the side effects of drugs such as digoxin. Potassium sparing diuretics tend to lead to hyperkalaemia.

Ceftazidime must be given in reduced doses even in mild renal impairment.

Allopurinol in renal failure is associated with increased toxicity and both the dose and frequency of administration should be decreased. Acyclovir worsens renal failure and must be given at a reduced dose.

Aronson JK. Drugs and Renal Insufficiency
Medicine 1999 27: 7; 113–118

Question 26

A. false **B.** false **C.** false **D.** false **E.** false

Absolute contraindications to thrombolysis with streptokinase are:

active internal bleeding
recent head trauma
intracranial tumour
CVA in last 2 months
uncontrolled hypertension (treat and then give)
previous administration of streptokinase

Relative contraindications are:

pregnancy
prolonged CPR
bleeding disorders
recent surgery
anticoagulation or an INR > 1.8
probable intracardiac thrombus

Holmberg SR. Thrombolysis in acute myocardial infarction
British Journal of Hospital Medicine 1992 47(8): 572–580

Question 27

A. false **B.** false **C.** true **D.** true **E.** false

If the initial serum iron concentration is 500 μg/l or more then the treatment is with desferrioxamine. The following are features of severe poisoning:

Vomiting
Diarrhoea
Convulsions
Coma
Hypotension
Hepatocellular failure
Renal failure
Cardiac failure
Hypovolaemic shock from haemorrhagic enterocolitis

Proudfoot A. Iron poisoning
Medicine 1999 27: 4; 40–42

Question 28

A. false **B.** true **C.** true **D.** true **E.** false

The incidence rate is the proportion of a defined group developing the condition within a stated period of time.

Prevalence is defined as the incidence × the average duration of the disease. Point prevalence is the proportion of a defined group having the condition at one point in time.

The mode is the most frequently occuring value.

The mean is the average of a set of values (sum of the values divided by the number of values).

The median is the middle value when they are arranged in order.

If a distribution is negatively skewed the mean is < median

If the distribution is positively skewed the mean is > median

The correlation coefficient is usually represented by r. It is a value between –1 and +1. The closer to zero it is the less the linear association is between 2 variables. A minus value of r means that as one variable goes down the other increases. A positive r value indicates that both values increase or decrease together.

The p value is the probability of observing a difference of that magnitude if the null hypothesis is true. A p value of 0.05 means there is a 1 in 20 chance that the difference occurred by chance alone.

The null hypothesis assumes there is no difference between the 2 populations being studied. A $p<0.01$ means the probability of the result occuring by chance is 1 in 100.

Driscoll P et al. Statistics 6: An introduction to hypothesis testing. Parametric comparison of two groups-1. J Accid Emerg Med 2001 18: 124–130

Driscoll P et al. Statistics 7: An introduction to hypothesis testing. Parametric comparison of two groups-2. J Accid Emerg Med 2001 18: 214–221

Question 29

A. false **B.** false **C.** true **D.** true **E.** false

Uveitis may present as an acute painful red eye or more insidiously with floaters, and loss of vision. Recurrent episodes lead to the development of cataracts, glaucoma, and permanent loss of vision. It accounts for 10% of patients registered blind under the age of 65. Uveitis is termed acute if it remits within 3 months of onset and chronic if it persists for longer. The majority of cases are idiopathic though it may occur with a variety of systemic diseases. All patients presenting with chronic uveitis should at least have a CXR, syphilis serology, and serum ACE performed. Treatment is with topical steroids initially, but resistant cases may need systemic steroids or other immunosuppressive agents.

Causes of uveitis include:

Ankylosing spondylitis
Behçets syndrome
Fungal infections
Inflammatory Bowel Disease (Crohn's > Ulcerative colitis)
Juvenile chronic arthritis
Lyme disease
Multiple sclerosis
Ocular Lymphoma
Retinoblastoma
Rheumatoid arthritis
Sarcoidosis
Syphilis
Tuberculosis
Vogt Koyanagi Harada syndrome (Neurological disorder comprising uveitis, deafness, and/or meningoencephalitis that occurs solely in oriental patients)

McCluskey PJ et al. Chronic uveitis
British Medical Journal. 2000 320(7234): 555–558

Question 30

A. true **B.** true **C.** true **D.** true **E.** false

The neurological effects of systemic lupus erythematosus (SLE) include

convulsions
aseptic meningitis
peripheral neuropathy
cranial nerve lesions

ataxia
hemiplegia/CVA
psychiatric conditions ranging from depression to schizophrenia

Hughes GRV Connective Tissue Diseases.
Third edition. Oxford: Blackwell Scientific Publications 1987

Schon NF. Neurology of systemic autoimmune disorders: a paediatric perspective
Semin Pediatr Neurol 2001 7: 2; 108–117

Question 31

A. false **B.** true **C.** false **D.** true **E.** true

Paget's disease is associated with increased bone turnover with increased osteoblastic and osteoclastic activity. There is an increase in alkaline phosphate and urinary hydroxyproline and a normal or slight increase in serum calcium. It is rare in the under 40's. The prevalence ranges from 4% over 40yrs to 10% of adults by age 90%. It is usually asymptomatic: less than 2% show symptoms.

Clinically patients may experience:

bone pain
high output cardiac failure
sarcoma
arthritis
skeletal deformity
fractures and pseudofractures
deafness, CN palsies and spinal stenosis secondary to nerve compression
hypercalcaemia if immobile

Treatment

bisphosphonates
calcitonin
mithramycin
surgery

A bone scan will show the extent of the disease with an increase in 'temperature' over the affected bone.

Ankrom MA, Shapiro JR. Paget's disease of bone (osteitis deformans)
Journal of the American geriatric society 1998 46(8): 1025–1033

Delmas PD, Meunier P Drug therapy: The management of Paget's disease of Bone
NEJM 1997 336(8): 558–566

Question 32

A. false **B.** true **C.** false **D.** false **E.** true

Mitral regurgitation and dilated cardiomyopathy both cause left ventricular dilatation which results in increased end diastolic dimension on echocardiograpny. Aortic stenosis and hypertrophic cardiomyopathy cause left venticular hypertrophy, not dilatation.

Echocardiographic features of left ventricular dysfunction:

1. LV enlargement
2. reduced fractional shortening
3. paradoxical septal motion
4. reduced EF slope
5. premature aortic valve closure or reduced valve opening

Causes of paradoxical septal motion:

1. congestive cardiomyopathy
2. ischaemic heart disease (infarction in the septum)
3. right ventricular overload eg secondary to an ASD
4. conduction disturbance eg LBBB, WPW
5. post surgical (CABG)

Features of mitral stenosis on echo:

1. thickened leaflets, calcification of the mitral valve
2. left atrial enlargement
3. atrial fibrillation (loss of a point)
4. poor excursion of the anterior leaflet
5. anterior position of the posterior leaflet throughout diastole said to be the most specific sign
6. reduced EF slope

Swanton RH. Cardiology 4th Ed. 1998. Blackwell Scientific Publications Ltd. Oxford

Question 33

A. true **B.** false **C.** true **D.** false **E.** false

Constrictive pericarditis usually results from pericardial fibrosis following haemorrhagic pericarditis. Causes include viral infections, tuberculosis, bacterial endocarditis, connective tissue disorders, malignancy, uraemia, drugs, and radiotherapy.

Patients usually present with signs of congestive cardiac failure in the absence of any history of angina or hypertension, and have a normal sized heart on CXR.

Clinically the JVP is elevated with a prominent x and y descent and a paradoxical rise in the JVP on inspiration may be present (Kussmaul's sign). The heart sounds are soft and there may be a ventricular knock causing a gallop rhythm. Atrial fibrillation is common. Hepatosplenomegaly, ascites, and peripheral oedema occur latterly.

Clinically differentiation from restrictive cardiomyopathy is extremely difficult. In restrictive cardiomyopathay the y descent in the JVP is absent, Kussmaul's sign is usually absent, and pulsus paradoxus is virtually always present.

In practice cardiac catheterization is used to differentiate between the two.

Swanton RH. Cardiology 4th Ed. 1998. Blackwell Scientific Publications Ltd. Oxford

Question 34

A. true **B.** false **C.** true **D.** true **E.** true

Eisenmenger's complex or syndrome refers to pulmonary hypertension secondary to increased pulmonary vascular resistance that causes a reversed, right to left shunt, most commonly through a large ventricular septal defect. Thus all cardiac defects that cause a right to left shunt give rise to Eisenmenger's syndrome.

An ostium secundum ASD is a relatively benign condition that is usually asymptomatic through childhood and adolescence. It is often an incidental diagnosis and generally does not cause symptoms until later life. Pulmonary hypertension and shunt reversal is rare and only occurs in adults.

For a further discussion of ASDs see Paper 1 question 32.

Fallots tetralogy classically refers to the combination of pulmonary stenosis, right ventricular hypertrophy, overriding of the aorta and a VSD. It is the commonest cause of cyanotic congenital heart disease in children. In the first 3–6 months of life the child is usually acyanotic though after this the shunt reverses giving the typical clinical picture. Squatting increases systemic vascular resistance reducing the right to left shunt and increasing pulmonary blood flow.

The ductus arteriosus allows blood to flow from the pulmonary artery into the aorta during fetal life. The duct usually closes in the first six weeks following birth. It is more likely to remain patent in premature babies. A left to right shunt then develops which if left untreated can ultimately cause pulmonary hypertension and shunt reversal.

Causes of a right to left shunt include

Ventricular septal defect
Atrial septal defect
A-V canal
Patent ductus arteriosus
Transposition of the great arteries
Hemi or total anomalous pulmonary venous drainage
Pulmonary atresia
Tricuspid atresia
Fallot's tetralogy

Swanton RH. Cardiology 4th Ed. 1998. Blackwell Scientific Publications Ltd. Oxford

Question 35

A. true **B.** false **C.** true **D.** false **E.** false

Coarctation of the aorta occurs distal to the left subclavian artery. Infantile forms arise before the ductus arteriosus, are associated with multiple other cardiac defects and present in the first few months of life with heart failure. In the adult form the coarctation is postductal and may not present until the 2nd or 3rd decade. Coarctation is associated with a bicuspid aortic valve (50–80% of cases), berry aneurysms, and Turner's and Noonan's syndromes. Aortic aneurysms and aortic dissections are also more common than in the general population.

In adults the diagnosis is usually made during investigation of hypertension, infective endocarditis, subarachnoid haemorrhage or following routine chest X-ray.

Older patients may present with heart failure secondary to valvular heart disease or with coronary artery disease. Physical signs may include upper limb hypertension, weak or absent femoral pulses, palpable collateral vessels, ejection systolic murmur, prominent carotid pulsations, and left ventricular hypertrophy. The coarctation itself may produce a loud systolic murmur best heard over the back. Rib notching and an abnormal or double aortic knuckle are seen on plain chest X-ray. The mainstay of treatment is reconstructive cardiac surgery with resection of the coarctation and re-anastomosis of the aorta. The coarctation may recur but is usually amenable to balloon dilatation. Bypass procedures using Dacron grafts may reduce the incidence of re-occurrence. In some centres balloon dilatation is replacing primary surgery though there are significant concerns regarding long-term patency.

All patients are at risk of bacterial endocarditis and require antibiotic prophylaxis for invasive procedures.

McCrindle BW. Coarctation of the aorta. Current opinion in Cardiology. 1999 14(5): 448–452

Question 36

A. false **B.** true **C.** true **D.** false **E.** false

Diseases that characteristically are of increasing severity and have an earlier age of onset with successive generations are said to display genetic anticipation. These disorders result from mutations that expand short repetitive segments of the genome beyond the normal range, normally around thirty repeats. These are called expanded triplet repeats and are mostly associated with neurodegenerative disorders.

Diseases that display genetic anticipation include:

Friedreich's ataxia
Huntington's chorea
Myotonic dystrophy (Steinert's disease)
Dentatorubropallidoluysian atrophy
Kennedy syndrome
Fragile X syndrome

For a discussion of myotonic dystrophy see Paper 5 question 37.

Question 37

A. true **B.** false **C.** false **D.** false **E.** true

Huntington's disease (HD) is an autosomal dominant disorder with a high degree of penetrance characterized by movement disorder, cognitive impairment, and emotional disturbance. It usually develops between 35 and 50 years though can appear at any age. It is a relentlessly progressive disorder with death occurring 15–20 years after the onset of symptoms. The movement disorder typically comprises involuntary choreiform movements along with a progressive disturbance of voluntary movement. In the late stages patients are mute and akinetic with severe rigidity and joint contractures. Cases that develop in childhood or adolescence are atypical, presenting with bradykinesia, rigidity and dystonia in the absence of chorea. Epilepsy and severe dementia is common in this group.

Cognitive impairment develops around the same time as the onset of physical symptoms though one symptom is usually predominant. Patients also commonly develop depression, irritability and apathy and there is a considerably raised suicide rate of around 12%.

The pathological basis for the disease is atrophy of the caudate nucleus and putamen (the corpus striatum within the basal ganglia). The HD gene is localised on chromosome 4. The gene was identified in 1993 with the mutation being a CAG trinucleotide repeat. Alleles with less than 36 triplets do not cause disease, alleles with 36–41 triplets are incompletely penetrant, with alleles longer than that always causing disease. The longer the repeat the earlier the onset of the disease (genetic anticipation). New mutations do occasionally occur. Diagnosis can now be made by direct gene testing of affected or at risk individuals.

Treatment is predominantly supportive as there are currently no therapies that slow progression of the disease. Neuroleptics eg haloperidol, thioridazine may be useful in managing movement disorders and dopamine depleting agents such as reserpine and tetrabenazine can be useful in treating resistant chorea though care must be taken as they can aggravate depression.

Dentatorubral-pallidoluysian atrophy is a related progressive neurological disorder seen predominantly in Japan with the same pattern of symptoms in adults.

Ross CA et al. Huntington Disease and the related disorder, Dentatorubral-Pallidoluysian Atrophy (DRPLA). Medicine. 1997 76(5): 305–338

Question 38

A. true **B.** true **C.** true **D.** true **E.** true

Causes of confusion and seizures in a patient with HIV include:

Infections:

CMV encephalitis
Toxoplasmosis
Cryptococcal meningitis
Tuberculous meningitis
Progressive multifocal leucoencephalitis

Drugs:

Nucleoside reverse transcriptase inhibitors eg zidovudine (AZT), zalcitabine (ddC)
Sodium Foscarnet

Miscellaneous:

HIV encephalopathy, Non-Hodgkin's lymphoma

For a discussion on the neurological sequelae of HIV infection see Paper 5 question 36.

Ledingham JGG, Warrell DA. Concise Oxford Textbook of Medicine 2000 Oxford University Press

Question 39

A. true **B.** true **C.** true **D.** false **E.** false

Central scotomata are blind spots indicative of intensive optic nerve damage. Unilateral scotoma may occur following optic nerve compression but bilateral scotoma generally indicate a hereditary, toxic or nutritional cause.

Causes of central scotomata include:

Optic neuritis: CMV, toxoplasmosis, rift valley fever, demyelination
Toxic amblyopia: alcohol, tobacco, methanol, lead
Nutritional amblyopia: vitamin B12 deficiency
Drugs: isoniazid, chlorpropamide, chloramphenicol, penicillamine
Pituitary tumours
Leber's optic atrophy
Macular degeneration

Ross Russel RW. Visual Pathways.
Oxford Textbook of Medicine. Oxford University Press.

Question 40

A. true **B.** true **C.** true **D.** false **E.** false

The following ECG changes are recognized in anorexia nervosa: sinus bradycardia, T-wave inversion and an increased QT interval.

Hoffman RS. Hall RC. Reversible EKG changes in anorexia nervosa. Psychiatric Medicine 1989 7(4): 211–216.

Question 41

A. false **B.** false **C.** false **D.** true **E.** true

Generally the chances of an aged depressed patient responding to treatment, whether ECT or antidepressant drugs is good, particularly if:

Biological symptoms are prominent

There is a record of a clear change in a patient's mood

There is a history of previous successful treatment

A family history of biological depression or mania

There is no clinical evidence of dementia from the history

There is less likely to be diurnal variation in symptoms of depression in the elderly than in the younger age group, but there is more likely to be associated physical disease in the older patients with depressive symptoms (depressive pseudodementia). Dementia-like symptoms of depression are very unusual except in the older age group.

A J D Macdonald. ABC of mental health: Mental health in old age. BMJ 1997 315: 413–417

Question 42

A. true **B.** true **C.** true **D.** true **E.** true

Wernicke's encephalopathy due to thiamine deficiency is commonly found in alcoholism, although it may appear in other syndromes of nutritional deficiency; it has been described in dialysis patients and hyperemesis gravidarum. There is often overlap between Wernicke's, the neurological disorder and Korsakoff's syndrome, which is psychiatric.

Features of Wernicke's encephalopathy

Neuronal loss in mamillary bodies
Associated lesions in and around the aqueduct and 4th ventricle
Lesions in the vermis and anterior cerebellar lobules

Opthalmoplegia
Nystagmus
Lateral rectus palsy
Horizontal conjugate gaze palsy
Cerebellar ataxia
Peripheral neuritis

Confusion
Apathy
Impaired awareness
Impaired concentration

Features of Korsakoff's syndrome

1. Loss of past memories
2. Inability to form new memories
3. Loss of insight
4. Confabulation (not always present for example may regress with disease progression).
5. Apathy
6. Limited response to thiamine due to severe neuropathology less than 25% make a full recovery.

Peters TJ. Physical complications of alcohol misuse. In Weatherall DJ, Ledingham JGG, Warrell DA, eds. Oxford Textbook of Medicine, Oxford: Oxford University Press, 1996

Question 43

A. false **B.** true **C.** false **D.** true **E.** true

Persecutory delusions and beliefs occur in severe depression. Third person auditory hallucinations, particularly in the third person as a commentary, thought insertion and somatic passivity are all part of Schneider's first rank symptoms of schizophrenia (see

Turner T. ABC of mental health: Schizophrenia. BMJ 1997 315: 108–111

Question 44

A. false **B.** false **C.** true **D.** false **E.** true

Peak flow meters, although cheap and easy to use are inaccurate, particularly at the extremes of low or high flow, but also in between patients, and with a high error at the mid-range also. They are highly dependent on patient effort, which seems to be particularly important in acute asthma, and when patients are unwell. Peak flows do not correlate well with FEV1 in cystic fibrosis, partly due to their inaccuracy, but also due to the nature of the disease. They are more useful when used as a measure of long-term response to treatment in individual patients. Predicted value scales all involve height to calculate expected peak flow.

Busse WW, Lemanske RF. Asthma: Advances in immunology
NEJM 2001 344: 5; 350–362

Hunt LW. How to treat difficult ashma cases. An action plan for physicians and patients
Postgrad Med 2001 109: 5; 61–68

Question 45

A. true **B.** false **C.** false **D.** false **E.** true

The associations of the above are detailed in Paper 2 Question 47.

Occupational causes of bronchogenic carcinoma:

Coal gas manufacture
Asbestos
Alpha radiation in mines, uranium exposure.
Polycyclic aromatics
Nickel
Chloromethyl ethers
Chromate
Arsenic processing

Epstein RJ. Medicine for examinations. 3rd Ed. Churchill Livingstone, London, 1996.

Patz EF et al. Screening for lung cancer
NEJM 2000 343: 22; 1627–1633

Question 46

A. true **B.** true **C.** false **D.** true **E.** true

Paper 3 Question 45 and Paper 5 Question 46 both give the explanations to this question.

Question 47

A. false **B.** false **C.** false **D.** true **E.** false

Asthma mortality in England and Wales is dropping by about 6% a year in people aged 5–64 years, and changing very slowly in the 65 years and over group despite its increasing prevalence. The downward trends in asthma mortality in Britain are probably due to increased use of prophylactic treatment.

Allergens from house dust mites are by far the most common allergen implicated in chronic allergic asthma, and furry pets are second most commonly implicated. Grass pollens are associated with seasonal symptoms.

Allergen immunotherapy, desensitization or hyposensitization has only been really successful in wasp and bee sting hypersensitivity. In fact the pollen and house-dust mite allergen extracts used for desensitisation have had poor results, with troublesome side effects, and even deaths due to anaphylaxis. Summer hay fever desensitization has been more successful.

The British Thoracic Society has published guidelines for asthma treatment in adults, which the candidate would do well at least to read before the exam. These have been referenced before in this book, and are also detailed in the British National Formulary. Inhaled corticosteroids are recommended in this situation; particularly as there has been much discussion over the last decade as to whether long-term use of beta 2 agonists increases the risk of morbidity and mortality from chronic allergic asthma.

Although high doses of inhaled corticosteroids used on a long term basis does increase the risk from osteoporosis, this should not deter one from using them in this group of patients. Standard recommendations about prophylaxis and monitoring for osteoporosis would of course apply.

M J Campbell, G R Cogman, S T Holgate, and S L Johnston.
Age specific trends in asthma mortality in England and Wales, 1983–95: results of an observational study.
BMJ 1997 314: 1439

Question 48

A. true **B.** true **C.** false **D.** true **E.** true

Small intestinal disorders causing malabsorption:

Coeliac disease
Dermatitis herpetiformis
Bacterial overgrowth
Intestinal resection/short bowel syndrome
Tropical sprue
Whipple's disease
Mesenteric vascular insufficiency
Radiation enteritis
Ileal Lymphoma
Parasite infestation
Giardia lamblia
Cryptosporidium
Drugs
Cholestyramine binds bile salts causing diarrhoea
Thyrotoxicosis
Zollinger-Ellison syndrome

Causes of Bacterial Overgrowth:

Intestinal stasis
Anatomic
Strictures
Diverticulosis
Surgery e.g. Jejuno-ileal bypass, Bilroth II
Motility disorders e.g. scleroderma

Abnormal connections between proximal and distal bowel
Fistulas
Ileocaecal valve disorders/resection

Hypochlorhydria
Chronic atrophic gastritis
Gastrectomy

Immunodeficiency
Primary
Acquired
Malnutrition

Age

Lead poisoning causes recurrent, often severe abdominal pain, oral ulceration, neuropathy and a metallic taste in the mouth. A gingival line may appear, with often anaemia and renal dysfunction. Diagnosis is established by urine testing over 72 hours.

Scheuner M, Yang H, Rotter JI. Malabsorption Disorders. In Yamada T, Alpers DH, Owyang C, Powell DW, Silverstein FE, eds. Textbook of Gastroenterology, Philadelphia: JB Lippincott Company, 1995

Question 49

A. false **B.** true **C.** true **D.** true **E.** false

Enteropathic arthritis, which is associated with ulcerative colitis is in the rheumatoid factor seronegative group. Likewise, ankylosing spondylitis and Reiters syndrome are both associated with UC whereas rheumatoid arthritis (RA) is not. Enteropathic synovitis occurs in 11% of patients with ulcerative colitis and although it is generally related to the activity of the underlying disease, may be the first manifestation of either the diagnosis of UC or an acute attack. Aetiology is unknown, although is likely to be related to immune-complex deposition. Ankylosing spondylitis, which is related to HLA B27 is present in about 5% of people with UC, a 30-fold increase compared to the normal population. Recently peripheral arthropathies without axial involvement in inflammatory bowel disease has been characterised and can be subdivided into a pauciarticular, large joint arthropathy and a bilateral polyarthropathy, each being distinguished by its articular distribution and natural history. Moreover there appears to be an HLA association for each of the subgroups. (See references).

Gastrointestinal manifestations of RA

1. temporomandibular joint involvement impeding chewing and causing nutritional impairment
2. sicca syndrome accompanied by stomatitis and gingivitis
3. oesophageal dysmotility
4. secondary amyloidosis involving the GI tract
5. vasculitis of mesenteric vessels causing intestinal ischaemia, bleeding and infarction.
6. cholecystitis, appendicitis, perisplenitis, splenic infarction, pancreatitis, and hepatic arteritis have been described
7. iatrogenic
   chronic administration of NSAIDs
   methotrexate causing hepatic fibrosis

Hepatic complications of IBD include fatty liver, pericholangitis, chronic active hepatitis, sclerosing cholangitis and ultimately cirrhosis. Pericholangitis is the most common hepatic complication of IBD with a prevalence as high as 80% reported in some studies. These patients are usually asymptomatic and elevations of Alkaline Phosphatase are often seen in IBD patients with no obvious cause. Sclerosing cholangitis occurs in up to 3–4% of patients with UC.

Acanthosis nigricans is localized hyperpigmentation of the neck, axillae, genital area and facial skin. It is associated with visceral malignancies such as stomach carcinomas, and lymphomas.

Stenson WF. Inflammatory Bowel Disease. In Yamada T, Alpers DH, Owyang C, Powell DW, Silverstein FE, eds. Textbook of Gastroenterology, Philadelphia: JB Lippincott Company, 1995

Orchard TR et al. Clinical phenotype is related to HLA genotype in the peripheral arthropathies in inflammtory bowel disease. Gastroenterology 2000 118 (2): 274–278.

Orchard TR et al. Peripheral arthropathies in inflammatory bowel disease: their articular distribution and natural history. Gut 1998 42(3): 387–391.

Question 50

A. true **B.** false **C.** false **D.** true **E.** false

Functional bowel disease or irritable bowel syndrome (IBS) forms a substantial proportion of the UK gastroenterology outpatient workload. It is estimated that it affects up to 15% of the adult population of the Western world at any one time, most of whom will not seek medical help. Whether the individuals who present to doctors have a different pathophysiological basis to their disease is unresolved.

The currently most-sited classification of functional bowel disease are the Rome Criteria, from the 13th international congress of Gastroenterology in 1990. Generally the term IBS describes the presence of abdominal pain associated with defecation, a change in bowel habit with disordered defecation with sometimes the sensation of abdominal distension.

The disease seems to be more common in women, and there are no specific endoscopic, radiological, pathological or physiological changes that can provide a positive diagnosis. Generally patients are investigated to exclude more sinister reasons for the symptoms, and in a careful history warning signs such as weight loss, rectal bleeding in a patient over the age of 40 and a short history are suggestive of alternative diagnoses such as a colonic carcinoma. The history typically extends for several years if not decades. Beware of diagnosing IBS in a patient with only a two week history. Women particularly with IBS complain of menstrual and bladder symptoms.

Thompson DG. Functional Bowel Disease and the Irritable Bowel Syndrome. In Weatherall DJ, Ledingham JGG, Warrell DA, eds. Oxford Textbook of Medicine, Oxford: Oxford University Press, 1996.

Horwitz BJ, Fisher RS. The Irritable Bowel Syndrome NEJM 2001 344: 24; 1846–1850

Question 51

A. false **B.** true **C.** false **D.** true **E.** true

Fulminant hepatic failure is usually defined as acute liver failure complicated by hepatic encephalopathy occurring within 8 weeks of the onset of clinical evidence of liver disease. The four principal manifestations are hepatocellular jaundice, hepatic encephalopathy, ascites and haemorrhagic diathesis (the prothrombin time is raised).

Some causes of fulminant hepatic failure:

Acute viral hepatitis (usually A and B)

Drug-induced:

Paracetamol
Halothane
Amanita mushrooms
Industrial solvents eg CCl_4

Vascular:

Budd-Chiari syndrome
Veno-occlusive disease may be induced by chemotherapy or irradiation

Autoimmune hepatitis

Wilson's disease

Precipitated by partial hepatectomy in the presence of cirrhosis

Acute fatty liver of pregnancy

Reye's syndrome

Heat stroke

Hepatocellular failure is associated with acid-base and electrolyte changes. Cerebral oedema and raised intracranial pressure are common. Hyponatraemia is common, with various causes, often due to the effects of the fluids given. Urinary sodium is often low, although not invariably so; patients are often given loop diuretics. Renal failure is common. As liver failure is associated with systemic vasodilation and hyperdynamic circulation, cardiac output is increased, pulmonary wedge pressure is increased and peripheral vascular resistance is decreased. Overall survival is only 20 to 25% with standard intensive medical care.

Jone EA. Hepatocellular failure. In Weatherall DJ, Ledingham JGG, Warrell DA, eds. Oxford Textbook of Medicine, Oxford: Oxford University Press, 1996.

Question 52

A. true **B.** true **C.** false **D.** true **E.** true

Hyperprolactinaemia is associated with hypogonadism, and/or galactorrhoea, and may indicate the presence of a pituitary adenoma or hypothalamic disease. Up to 40% of women with amenorrhoea have hyperprolactinaemia, and about 30% of women with amenorrhoea and galactorrhoea have prolactin-secreting pituitary tumours. The functional hypogonadism in women can be regarded in part as a desirable physiologic mechanism whereby breast-feeding causes decreased fertility and delayed resumption of menses.

Hyperprolactinaemia in men can cause impotence and infertility; with prolactin excess FSG and LH levels in men decline and serum testosterone drops.

Causes of hyperprolactinaemia:

Physiological:

Pregnancy
Nursing
Stress
Sleep
Food ingestion

Drugs:

Dopamine receptor antagonists
E.g. Phenothiazines
Dopamine-depleting agents
E.g. Methyldopa
Oestrogens
Opiates

Disease:

Pituitary tumours
Hypothalamic and pituitary stalk disease
Primary hypothyroidism
Chronic renal failure
Cirrhosis
Chest wall trauma
Seizures

Daniels GH, Martin JB. Neuroendocrine Regulation and Diseases of the Anterior Pituitary and Hypothalamus. In Isselbacher KJ, Braunwald E, Wilson JD et al., eds. Harrisons Principles of Internal Medicine, 13th Edition. New York: McGraw-Hill, 1994.

Question 53

A. true **B.** true **C.** false **D.** true **E.** false

Anterior pituitary hormone deficiencies

Total or selective hypopituitarism may occur in patients with pituitary adenomas, parasellar diseases, following pituitary surgery or radiation (including cranial radiation for intracranial malignancies), or following head injury (see list below). Deficiency of any or all of the six major hormones secreted by the pituitary can occur. A fall in/or cessation of gonadal function is the most common symptom in both men and women. Secondary hypogonadism may result from LH and FSH deficiency, but may also occur with hyperprolactinaemia. The classic finding is progressive loss of pituitary hormone secretion in the following order: gonadotrophin (LH, FSH), GH, TSH, ACTH, but, variations occur and some patients may have ACTH and/or TSH deficiency as the initial presenting feature. Prolactin deficiency is uncommon and is usually caused by pituitary infarction. The most common presentation is cessation of growth or delayed puberty in children.

Causes of hypopituitarism:

Isolated hormone deficiencies:
Congenital or acquired deficiencies

Tumours:

pituitary adenomas
pituitary apoplexy
hypothalamic tumours e.g. craniopharyngiomas
metastatic carcinoma

Inflammatory diseases:

granulomatous disease sarcoid, tuberculosis
eosinophilic granuloma

Vascular disease:

Sheehan's postpartum necrosis

Destructive or traumatic events:

surgery
radiation
trauma

Infiltration:

haemochromatosis
amyloid

Autoimmune disease

ACTH deficiency results in cortisol deficiency, manifested by fatigue, decreased appetite, weight loss, decreased pigmentation, abnormal response to stress characterized by fever hypotension, hyponatraemia and a reduced plasma cortisol response to insulin-induced hypoglycaemia. Unlike primary adrenal deficiency ACTH deficiency does not cause hyperpigmentation, hyperkalaemia or salt loss. Due to the normal diurnal variation in cortisol, the morning is the most reliable time to take a level. At night the normal range approaches the limit of detection by routine methods.

A short Synacthen (SYNthetic ACTHen) test is a good screening test and involves giving 0.25mg synthetic ACTH, measuring cortisol levels prior to the test and at 30 and 60 minutes post injection. Low values of cortisol are consistent with either primary or secondary hypoadrenalism. Patients with secondary hypoadrenalism in the longer Synacthen test, involving 1mg of depot Synacthen, will show higher values of cortisol over succeeding days due to recruitment of adrenal function by the continued supply of ACTH. Patients with primary adrenal dysfunction will show no response.

Thorner MO. Anterior pituitary disorders. In Weatherall DJ, Ledingham JGG, Warrell DA, eds. Oxford Textbook of Medicine, Oxford: Oxford University Press, 1996.

Question 54

A. true **B.** true **C.** true **D.** false **E.** false

In the blood T4 and T3 are almost entirely bound to plasma-proteins. T4 is bound, in order of frequency, to thyroxine-binding globulin (TBG), to a T4-binding prealbumin and to albumin. However only the free, unbound hormone is available to tissues. The total serum thyroxine is the laboratory measurement of free and bound T4, and is therefore primarily related to the concentration of binding plasma-proteins. Decreases and increases of TBG will cause a reduced or increased total serum T4 respectively, at least acutely before the concentration of free T4 is altered to maintain homeostasis. These are the causes of alterations in the serum TBG:

Increased:

Pregnancy, oestrogens, OCP
Hereditary
Phenothiazines, perphenazine, clofibrate
Viral hepatitis
Acute intermittent porphyria
Myxoedema

Decreased:

Hereditary
Androgens, asparaginase
Corticosteroids, anabolic steroids
Active acromegaly
Nephrotic syndrome
Malnutrition
Major illness, surgery
Thyrotoxicosis

De Quervains thyroiditis, also known as subacute, granulomatous, giant-cell or acute non-suppurative thyroiditis is due to a viral infection of the thyroid gland, and is associated with an acutely tender painful thyroid enlargement with constitutional features including fever, sweating, high a ESR. It most commonly affects young women and may start insidiously with features of an upper respiratory infection. Mononuclear cell infiltration of follicles with follicular disruption and loss of colloid are characteristic and may be confused with autoimmune thyroiditis. The disease usually affects the thyroid bilaterally although may be unilateral. Painful dysphagia is common. Symptoms and signs of hyperthyroidism may be present, although not invariably and there is characteristically a low or absent thyroidal uptake of radioactive iodine. In the acute stage the follicular changes progress to granuloma formation, and follicular destruction leads to release of preformed thyroxine but the synthesis of new hormone is inhibited. Notice from the question stem *characteristic* features are requested and therefore stem d) is false however once stores of preformed hormone are depleted, clinical and biochemical evidence of hypothyroidism may follow. Ultimately thyroid function returns to normal.

McGregor AM. The thyroid gland and disorders of thyroid function. In Weatherall DJ, Ledingham JGG, Warrell DA, eds. Oxford Textbook of Medicine, Oxford: Oxford University Press, 1996.

Question 55

A. true **B.** true **C.** true **D.** false **E.** true

Diabetic neuropathy may affect any part of the nervous system with the possible exception of the brain. Distinct syndromes can be recognized and several different types are often manifest in the same patient.

1. Peripheral polyneuropathy is the most common picture. Usually bilateral, the symptoms include numbness, paraesthesia, severe

hyperaesthesia and pain. Involvement of proprioceptive fibres leads to abnormalities of gait and development of Charcot's joints. Loss of vibratory sense is a typical examination finding, and is often an early development.

2. Mononeuropathy is less common. Characteristically there is sudden wrist drop, foot drop or paralysis of the cranial nerves III, IV or VI, cranial nerves, causing diplopia. Mononeuropathy is characterised by a high degree of spontaneous reversibility often over a several-week period.
3. Radiculopathy is a sensory syndrome in which pain occurs over the distribution of one or more spinal nerves, usually in the chest or abdomen. Severe pain may mimic herpes zoster or acute abdomen.
4. Autonomic neuropathy presents in a number of ways including ejaculatory failure. The gastrointestinal tract is a prime target, with dysphagia, delayed gastric emptying or alteration of bowel habit. Erectile dysfunction is said to be associated with a failure of nitric oxide generation in the penile vasculature.
5. Diabetic amyotrophy is probably due to neuropathy, although it may resemble primary muscle disease. Atrophy and weakness of the large muscles of the leg and pelvic girdle are often accompanied by anorexia and depression. Weight loss can be profound.

Myotonia is the repetitive depolarisation of muscle cells causing muscle contraction and is found in myotonic dystrophy and myotonia congenita. It is not a feature of diabetic neuropathy.

Types of diabetic tissue damage:

Microangiopathy (particularly retina, kidneys)
Macroangiopathy (accelerated arteriosclerosis (distally), e.g. ischaemic heart disease, cerebrovascular disease, intermittent claudication or gangrene of feet)
Neuropathy (autonomic, sensory, motor)
Ocular cataracts
Inelastic collagen (e.g. Dupuytren's contractures)

Marsden CD. Metabolic and deficiency disorders of the nervous system. In Weatherall DJ, Ledingham JGG, Warrell DA, eds. Oxford Textbook of Medicine, Oxford: Oxford University Press, 1996.

Question 56

A. true **B.** true **C.** false **D.** false **E.** true

See Paper 6 Question 56.

Question 57

A. false **B.** false **C.** true **D.** false **E.** true

Renal papillary necrosis can present acutely with haematuria, severe pyelonephritis and septicaemia, and renal failure, or subacutely with recurrent urinary tract infections and intermittent renal colic. Modest proteinuria is usually present (<2g/24hr). The necrotic papillae may remain in situ causing chronic interstitial nephritis, or slough leading to renal colic and ureteric obstruction.

Causes include diabetes mellitus, sickle cell anaemia, analgesic nephropathy, and tuberculosis.

Barnes DJ, Pinto JR, Viberti GC. The patient with diabetes mellitus. Davidson MA et al. Oxford Textbook of Clinical Nephrology. 2nd Ed. 1998. Oxford University Press. Oxford.

Question 58

A. false **B.** true **C.** true **D.** false **E.** false

Normal individuals excrete 1.5–20 µg/min of albumin whilst urinary dipsticks do not detect protein excretion of <200 µg/ min. Thus microalbuminuria refers to the subclinical range of excess albumin excretion between 20 and 200 µg/min. It is detected by radio-immunoassay. Albumin excretion shows a diurnal variation so the diagnosis of microalbuminuria needs to be based on at least three separate samples.

Microalbuminuria is predictive of early death, coronary artery disease, retinopathy, neuropathy, and peripheral vascular disease as well as frank proteinuria and progressive nephropathy. It is usually associated with hypertension, and raised cholesterol and triglyceride concentrations. The GFR is elevated at this stage but begins to fall with the onset of clinical proteinuria. Tight glycaemic control is mandatory and delays progression to overt nephropathy. ACE inhibitors also delay progression of diabetic nephropathy and should be used as first line agents in hypertensive subjects. Smoking is also associated with microalbuminuria and patients should be strongly advised to give up.

Viberti G. Diabetic Nephropathy
Medicine 1997 25(7): 32–35

Question 59

A. true **B.** false **C.** true **D.** false **E.** true

Normal protein excretion is <150mg/24hrs. There are three ways this can be exceeded leading to the development of proteinuria.

1. Glomerular basement membrane filter becomes increasingly porous. Eg the glomerulonephritides
2. Increased plasma concentration of circulating protein means filtered load exceeds reabsorptive capacity of the kidney. Eg albumin infusion, Bence-Jones proteinuria, lysozyme excretion in myelomonocytic leukaemia.
3. Proximal tubular damage impairs reabsorptive ability of kidney. Eg Fanconi syndrome

Proteinuria of up to 1.5–2g/day may be caused by any of these processes but anything in excess must be glomerular in origin. Glomerular proteinuria may range up to 100g/24hrs in exceptional cases.

Renal vein thrombosis occurs as a consequence of the hypercoagulable state that develops in the nephrotic syndrome. It is clinically apparent in up to 10% of cases of membranous nephropathy, and 2–3% of other glomerulonephritides. Sub clinical thrombosis as demonstrated by venography is present in a considerably higher proportion of cases.

Cameron JS. The patient with proteinuria and/or haematuria.
Davidson MA et al. Oxford Textbook of Clinical Nephrology. 2nd Ed. 1998.
Oxford University Press. Oxford.

Question 60

A. true **B.** false **C.** false **D.** false **E.** false

Rapidly progressive proliferative glomerulonephritis is defined histologically on the basis of crescent formation. Thus it is the only diagnostic feature. The rest of the features are present but are not diagnostic.

For further discussion see Paper 2 question 57.

Index Answers

Appendix

Membership and the Web

Introduction

As estimates of doctors who do not use the Internet range from 50 to 65% it is likely that this introductory article on the subject will be helpful for at least some of the candidates taking the exam. Medicine and exams are changing fast – the removal of negative marking from May 2002 for the MRCP I exam is a case in point. It goes without saying that the Internet and medical sites available on it are also changing, and part of this is the way computers are affecting the process. In Portsmouth hospital for example there are two monitors with independent Internet access on every ward. In St Vincent's Hospital, Sydney in addition to internet and intranet access certain general medical wards have full digital access to X-rays including CT scans minutes after the investigation has been undertaken with fully typed and signed radiology reports following 1–2hrs later, though hard copies of films are still preferable. For those studying for the MRCP exam if you look hard there are many textbooks, and many journals available for free on the Internet. In the UK and Australia hospital libraries provide access to a number of core *online* medical journals: some of these journals can be accessed from your home if you go through the library web site. There are sites available where you could do MRCP I MCQ's on any hospital based computers, practically any time of day or night if you wanted to.

Whole books and journals exist concerning medicine and the Internet; this article however is meant only to be an introduction to the subject for those new to the medium. With a little bit of reading and searching after reading this you should be able to research good peer reviewed medical sites that can contribute to your MRCP study. The article is aimed at those starting out but hopefully will have something to offer even to those who are well versed in medicine on the Internet. Do let us know if you have any suggestions or new sites, and we will incorporate them into the next edition. Skip the 'getting started' bit if you already have a computer and are already connected to the Internet.

A word of caution: computers are great time wasters! In addition to MRCP 'widows and widowers' the equivalent group for computers also exist. This exam is about doing as many MCQs as you can with access to good focussed annotations as answers; whilst this article has many key sites to studying to pass Part 1 MRCP there are many sites of general interest. Don't let your attention slide onto them for too long. (They can always be viewed after the exam!).

This article will be on the CD-ROM available with the book: it will be available as a Microsoft Word file and also in 'rich text format' in order that you may click on the links directly without typing them into your browser. An alternative is to copy and paste the links into your browser. Links that you find useful can then be copied into your 'favourites' folder within your browser. Remember that sites change all the time – the Royal College of Physicians is a good example of this – as they are upgraded and improved further, the addresses or 'Url's may change. If an address does not work try entering a search for the site using Google.

Getting Started

Hardware & Software

It is beyond the scope of this book to go into computer specifics and hardware but suffice to say that desktops and laptops are progressing in their specification every month and generally are becoming cheaper. Despite what you may read or hear, in fact, for this book and the majority of Internet use a relatively basic computer is all you need, so long as it is set up for the Internet. Any computer store will advise you on the current specifications for 'mid range priced computers' that are 'internet ready' – i.e. come complete with a modem (allowing you to access the internet with your telephone) and software to be able to access the internet ('browsers'). For each hospital within every medical directorate there is usually *someone* who is computer literate who can advise you on what to buy. Really expensive machines are required for software containing fast graphics such as computer games. For searching the internet, word processing, preparing slides for grand rounds, searching MEDLINE for their research papers undertaken after the MRCP exam then a computer in the mid range price bracket will be totally adequate and so long as there is the room to upgrade may last you well into the next 3–5 years. If a computer is being bought from scratch then there are many offers in terms of excellent business suite softwares e.g. Microsoft Office & Lotus SmartSuite, and hardware such as printers that may be bundled with it. If you are taking the plunge for the first time it pays to shop around, talk to colleagues at work, and cut out adverts of interest from the computer magazines, place them side by side in order to compare prices, specifications and – important when starting out for the first time – after sales help such as help desks and servicing.

Internet Service Providers (ISPs)

Are the next step. They give you an account to enable you to use your web browser and an email address. There are hundreds to choose from, and it is worth choosing carefully as once you sign up it may be arduous to have to change your email address.

Acrobat Reader

This is the program that allows you to read full text online, as a pdf. document. You can download it for free, either from

http://www.adobe.com/

or from the site you are trying to download the program from. Acrobat reader is generally a read only medium, and is ideal for printing. Text and graphics tools are available to copy relevant sections from any article (cf copyright).

Surfing the Internet

Many directories exist to allow the user to 'surf' the Internet for medical sites.

A directory is a large listing of web sites (listed hierarchically). The Yahoo web site is a good example of this and one of the best-known directories.

http://www.yahoo.com/

It is not itself a search engine but a directory for broad categories. With the use of directories it is relatively easy to get to subject gateways which contain a list of links to certain resources within a given subject area. You should regard these gateways as catalogues. Examples of some 'gateways' are the following:

Subject Gateways

Medical Matrix

http://www.medmatrix.org

This is a collection of medical sites all evaluated by physicians/clinicians and medical librarians. Once you have registered (free) you will have access to a comprehensive database of medical web sites both for patients and clinicians.

Yahoo Health

http://dir.yahoo.com/Health

Omni – organizing medical networked information

http://omni.ac.uk

BUBL link – medical sciences, medicine

http://link.bubl.ac.uk/medicine/

Search Engines on the Internet

Search engines search for specific text on the Internet on web pages. Generally they load very quickly and give results promptly. If you are unsuccessful with one then it may be worth trying others. Good examples of these are:

Google

http://www.google.com

Try putting in MRCP and see what happens.

Alta Vista

http://uk.altavista.com/

Northern Light

http://www.northernlight.com

Search engines specific for medicine:

Med Hunt

http://www.hon.ch/MedHunt/

Medical World Search

http://www.mwsearch.com

This requires registration and subscription.

In general search engines will only be able to search for text on open web sites. Sites that are within the medical literature often do not come up such as medical journals; for these you need to use dedicated databases specific for those areas of interest such as PubMed or Ovid for Medline, or the Cochrane database. Many of the sites listed in such a search are 'subscription only'.

Databases

PubMed (Medline)

http://www.ncbi.nlm.nih.gov/PubMed/

PubMed, a service of the National Library of Medicine, is also popular for Medline. Publishers participating in PubMed electronically supply NLM with their citations prior to or at the time of publication. There is free access to all abstracts from this searchable bibliographic database of records dating back to 1966. If the publisher has a web site that offers full-text of its journals, PubMed provides links to that site, as well as sites to other biological data, sequence centres etc. PubMed also has a list of all journals that are currently allowing free full-text access though you may need to try these through your postgraduate library, on site within your hospital.

Current Medline Scanner

http://bioinformatics.weizmann.ac.il/cms

CMS at the time of press was currently inoperative pending repairs to make it compatible with the new PubMed format.

Pub Crawler

http://www.gen.tcd.ie/pubcrawler/

A free update alerting service that scans the daily updates to PubMed and GenBank databases for topics of your choice.

Web Resources for MRCP

When first researching this subject we expected to find lots of free resources on the Internet, with questions and answers, and interactive facilities. In fact the range is quite restricted, possibly related to the relatively few people who are taking the exam.

Sites specific to MRCP

A good place to start is the Royal College site itself,

http://www.rcplondon.ac.uk

This is the main web site for the Royal College, and is fairly typical of sites like it. Informative, but with little of real interest to 'focussed' MRCP Part 1 candidates. Go straight to:

http://www.mrcpuk.org/

This is the main site for the examination. It contains application forms for the exam, an online version of the exam handbook, with examination regulations, and information for candidates, including dates, last possible application date and fees. The site contains order forms for MRCP publications, but as yet there are no plans to put results online. The site doesn't contain questions, clinical information or exam advice. For those new to browsing the Internet it should be noted that this site is extremely well put together: that said, it may not be entirely obvious how the site works. For example to see if a 'link' exists it is often useful to hold your cursor over some text and see if it changes to another cursor/icon such as a 'hand' in Internet Explorer'. Try putting your cursor over the word 'Menu' – then when the list appears place the cursor over 'MRCP UK' – here an arrow to the right of the text indicates that a list is available off this submenu. To go to any link simply click over any given text that provides that link. From the main web site, http://www.rcplondon.ac.uk it is possible to gain access to the following master class:

http://www.rcplondon.ac.uk/college/edu/edu[rule]medicalmasterclass.htm

Medical Masterclass is a modular distance learning education publication to support those intending to sit the MRCP (UK) examination (parts 1 and 2). It is edited by Dr John Firth, Addenbrooke's Hospital, Cambridge, UK, and contains 12 modules and 2 CD-ROMs with additional interactive case-scenarios and a dedicated web site with regular updates, case-scenarios, links to relevant reviews or papers and self-assessment questions. For some the medical masterclass may be expensive, at about £500, but may become essential effectively for anyone taking the exam. The web site will only be available to members with the appropriate passwords. If many candidates are sitting the exam would your postgraduate department consider getting an institutional license?

Many courses exist for studying the exam. Many of these courses have their own web sites though of course you may only have access to their own material.

PasTest

http://www.pastest.co.uk

Contains information about the books, courses and software, you can buy things from the site, and there is a small 'links section'. There is a question section, but it is only available to people who have done a course.

MRCP.Com

http://www.mrcp.com

and

http://www.onexamination.com/site/regInfo.asp

The team behind www.onExamination.com and MRCP.com are 7 British doctors who have formed 'Medelect Limited'. You have to pay to register and have access to the site, but it does look useful; and could be used as a centre from which to plan your studies. There are about 1500 questions, and the site remembers your scores for the next time. There is a book review site; but again, as with other training sites there is a reluctance to recommend competitor products. This site provides an MRCP 'course finder' and constantly reminds you how many days it is to the next exam! In terms of questions for money £30 for six months may seem quite expensive, but it isn't expensive compared to the drudgery and costs of a retake.

MCQs.com

http://www.mcqs.com

This site allows you to register for various exams questions and costs $25 for MRCP. It seems to be run from Malta, to find out how many questions are available you have to sign up for the site. Good information about the site is available at: *http://mcqs.com/new/about.htm*

Appendix

An article like this would not be complete without listing the publisher's website:

Greenwich Medical Media

http://www.greenwich-medical.co.uk/

Follow the links

Books > Category: General Medicine and Infectious Diseases > Q Notes for the MRCP I!

Other medical sites that might help

Although these sites are not specific to MRCP they provide centres from which you can access many other resources on the web.

http://www.doctors.net.uk

It is the most popular medical site in Europe with 50,000 members. It can be used as your ISP, or just a mobile email service (as mentioned above it is available from any ward in my hospital) and has the added benefit of making it look like you are doing something medical on the ward while accessing your email! Access is free once you register with your GMC number. Services include the 'journalert', where you can be emailed each week when papers are published on journals of your choice, Medline access, and free offers on books and equipment. The bulletin boards provide a forum for discussion and not surprisingly Membership is a common subject.

http://www.medix-uk.com

Actually quite similar to Doctors.net with a range of services. Like Doctors.net you need your GMC number to register but you only need to do it once.

http://www.mdlinx.com/

MDLinx is a network of nearly 40 specialty Web sites for physicians and healthcare professionals. The company is designed to provide physicians with a comprehensive one-stop site in each specialty, that delivers the 'focused information doctors need to stay current, deliver better care, and stay ahead of their patients.' It is designed as a 'one-stop resource' for physicians. You can use the link above to access the sites on most of the specialties, medical and surgical. The sites are pretty good, and visits are worthwhile if there is something you are interested in. They are all free though registration is required. Generally many features are news-orientated.

http://omni.ac.uk

Omni contains speciality pages, which all contain links to other interesting, or valuable sites related to that speciality. They are all evaluated for content. Look out for the free "teach yourself" tutorial on Internet information skills for medics.

Emergency Medicine

http://www.emedicine.com/

This colourful, interesting and well-funded site is a big site in every sense of the word. It contains one of the world's largest collections of medical reviews available on the Internet and currently it remains free for most articles. Full size pictures require an annual subscription of around $20 US (to defray costs of providing this service free to the third world). There is an excellent search engine and a good tutorial on how to get the best out of the site. For example: type 'fibrosing alveolitis' into the search engine at the top left hand side of the opening page. For every subject you are given the choice of selecting which emphasis you want the article to come under e.g. consumer/patient or professional. After these are selected or deselected press the 'Find Articles' button at the bottom of the page or simply select the choose articles at the top that have been selected by the search engine. In this case select: 'Pulmonary Fibrosis, Idiopathic' first by holding your cursor over the subject for a synopsis then by clicking on the text. A short read of this article will demonstrate how useful a site such as this will be for emergency internal medicine and the exam.

Medicine Online

http://www.meds.com/

This is a colourful site and free, although it requires registration. There are many links to other sites; advertising itself as "offering medical information and education in oncology and HIV/AIDS, Medline literature searches, Daily Medical News, Cancer Forums discussion groups, and reports from medical meetings for health care professionals, patients, and other interested consumers."

Search Sites

This is slightly outside the remit of this article. Although in general doing as many MCQs as you can is the best advice, there will come a time when you need to look things up. Both Doctors.net and Medix have access to textbooks, which are easy to use.

Otherwise Medline could be used e.g. through the BMA Medline service if you are a member: *http://ovid.bma.org.uk*

Otherwise BioMedNet:

http://www.biomednet.com/db/medline

which is free, and has a facility to let you download onto reference management programs, like Reference Manager, or ProCite.

Appendix

Entrez PubMed

http://www.ncbi.nlm.nih.gov/PubMed/

As discussed above.

Journal Sites

These are all self-explanatory. Although many have full text available only on subscription, you may be able to get full text access via your hospital postgraduate library. Most journal sites have excellent search engines, both for the journal itself, and beyond. Equally many of the search engines can be used without having to log in and results of searches will be available in abstract format.

British Medical Journal

http://www.bmj.com

Full text available for free. An excellent site, with added material compared to the paper edition.

New England Journal of Medicine

http://content.nejm.org/

Full text available with subscription. The NEJM has a useful service which emails you the contents each week automatically. There is an excellent search engine and collection of reviews which can be accessed immediately from the opening page of the web site ('15 most recent review articles').

The Lancet

http://www.thelancet.com/

An attractive site, with nice pictures, which doesn't take long to load. Full text available only on subscription. Registration without payment will give you restricted access to the search engine and free articles.

Postgraduate Medical Journal

http://www.postgradmedj.com/

Full text on subscription. The opening page has a good example of the availability on occasion of free articles such as the 'Editor's Choice.'

Hospital Medicine

http://www.hospitalmedicine.co.uk/

Full text available on line with subscription.

Hospital Practice

http://www.hosppract.com/index.htm

Although there is free full text the journal suspended publication in September 2001. Follow the link to 'Past Articles' to some useful general medical reviews.

Journal of the American Medical Association

http://jama.ama-assn.org/

Full text on subscription.

Evidence-Based Medicine

http://www.acponline.org/journals/ebm/sepoct99/ebmsomenu.htm

http://ebm.bmjjournals.com/

Evidence-Based Medicine is a co-publication of the BMJ Publishing Group and the American College of Physicians-American Society of Internal Medicine. Full text on subscription.

Internet Journal of Internal Medicine

http://www.ispub.com/journals/IJIM/current.htm

The Internet Journal of Internal Medicine is free and has a good search engine. Going to the home page of the internet publishers *http://www.ispub.com/* will provide links to the other journals that are available (follow the links for 'eJournals') to get to: *http://www.ispub.com/ejournals.htm*.

Recent articles of interest

1. Ward JP. Gordon J. Field MJ. Lehmann HP. Communication and information technology in medical education.

Lancet 357(9258): 792–6, 2001

Available free, this is a useful review, describing how medical schools are rising to the challenge of integrating the ways in which communication and information technology can be used to enhance the learning and teaching environment, and discuss the potential impact of future developments on medical education. The article contains links to other useful sites also.

2. Gorman PJ. Meier AH. Rawn C. Krummel TM. The future of medical education is no longer blood and guts, it is bits and bytes.

American Journal of Surgery 180(5): 353–6, 2000.

Another review article that looks at the future of the Internet, computing and medicine, from an American point of view.

3. Mehta N. Searching the Internet for medical information: practical tips.

Cleveland Clinic Journal of Medicine 66(9): 543–6, 549–50, 553, 1999.

This many not be readily available (it's not on the internet, but your library will be able to get hold of a copy).

4. Church RD. Elves AW. Inman R. Scriven PM. Using the Internet for postgraduate medical education.

Hospital Medicine (London) 60(5): 370–1, 1999

Other Speciality Resources:

Below is a list of various speciality-specific sites. As the sites become upgraded the addresses may change. It may be worth putting in a broad term for the main search title into a search engine such as 'Google' for example 'Endocrinology' and see what comes up.

Gastroenterology

http://www.gastrohep.com

GastroHep.com is a new site from Roy Pounder, Royal Free Hospital, London. An excellent gastroenterology resource, well designed, fully sponsored, with links to articles, journals (although of course not the full text of most) and general news. Subscription is free for a short time, and Eisai/Janssen-Cilag are sponsoring subscriptions at present, but ultimately will cost £65 per year.

Gastro Web

http://www.gastroweb.co.uk

The AstraZeneca-sponsored web site is good too, and is free, but you'll need your GMC number. It contains access to lecture slides on GI disease, Feldman's GI Atlas, PubMed, Reuters Health and a conference calendar.

Medscape

http://www.medscape.com/px/urlinfo

Medscape is an excellent website for many of the medical specialities and gastroenterology is well represented here.

http://www.medscape.com/Home/Topics/gastroenterology/gastroenterology.html

The site includes gastroenterology resources for clinicians, medical students and nurses as well as for patients.

Other sites:

http://www.gilinx.com

Requires registration

Cardiology

http://www.ecglibrary.com/ecghome.html

and

http://www.arrhythmiaonline.com

These are both free online libraries of ECGs. The second requires registration.

http://www.medtronic.com/OPTseries/index.jsp

The Online Presentation Tools web site (OPTseries.com) is a presentation resource. This is primarily cardiology-based; you need to register but it is free. It contains treatment guidelines, presentation tools, and a cardiology photo library. There is an emphasis towards American practice.

http://www.merck.com/product/usa/aggrastat/hcp/home.html

A site produced by MSD; in addition to the drug and trial information, it contains useful educational tools such as videos and presentations.

British Cardiological Society

http://www.bcs.com/

This is the home page of the British Cardiological Society.

Endocrinology

http://www.endo-direct.com/

ENDO Direct is Internet resource providing information on new developments in endocrinology. It provides access to full-text articles (only available to subscribers) from selected journals. There is also free access to review articles and special issues from these journals. The site has a calendar of events and a list of related links.

http://www.medther.gla.ac.uk/sites/endocrin.html

This gives quite a good list of links to endocrinology sites.

http://www.umds.ac.uk/elsewhere/physiology/banks/endorep.html£start

This probably stands out; it is an educational lecture series that offers briefs on hormones, the pituitary and hypothalamus, the thyroid gland, the adrenal gland, sex hormones and reproduction, etc. Produced by St. Thomas's Hospital for dentists.

http://www.diabetes.org.uk/home.htm

Diabetes UK is the new name for the British Diabetic Association. It is a good site with plenty of information and links, although nothing specific for the MRCP exam.

Respiratory Medicine:

http://www.chestnet.org/

This is the site of the American College of Chest Physicians. It contains a few more links, although, again, nothing specific for the MRCP exam.

http://www.medmark.org/rm/rm2.html

This site contains an enormous list of chest links. For example it can be used as a springboard for searches for guidelines etc.

Neurology

http://www.theabn.org/

The web site of the Association of British Neurologists; contains more information and links, with some career advice.

Pharmacology

The BNF

http://www.bnf.org

Says exactly what it does on the tin. The Internet version of the BNF. Good search engines, easy to understand and read, etc. Look it up on the ward when you can't find the paper one.

http://www.bps.ac.uk/BPS.html

The home page of the British Pharmacological Society. Provides a directory of educational teaching and learning resources.

http://sis.nlm.nih.gov/Chem/ChemMain.html

Chemical and drug information files held at the Division of Specialized information Services at the National Library of Medicine.

Nephrology

http://www.kidneyatlas.org/

This online edition of "Atlas of Diseases of the Kidney" series edited by Robert W. Schrier, Professor of Medicine, University of Colorado School of Medicine, is made available on the Web sponsorship. Has more than 2500 images, schematics, tables and algorithms. This publication is aimed at nephrologists, transplant surgeons and hypertension specialists, but may well be of use to you.

Emergency Medicine

http://www.bestbets.org/

'Best Evidence Topics' or BETs were developed in the Emergency Department of Manchester Royal Infirmary, UK, to provide rapid evidence-based answers to real-life clinical questions, using a systematic approach to reviewing the literature. BETs are intended to take into account the shortcomings of current evidence, allowing physicians to make the best of what there is. Has quite good search and browse facilities, and allows you to put your own questions.

http://www.emjonline.com/

The Emergency Medicine Journal (formerly the Journal of Accident and Emergency Medicine) covers developments within the field of emergency medicine, including all specialities involved in emergency care, such as acute medicine, intensive care, elderly care, surgery, paediatrics, psychiatry, trauma, pre-hospital care, and toxicology. Published by the BMJ Publishing Group. Full text available on line with subscription.

http://www.embbs.com/aem/aemweb.html

A collection of case studies with accompanying photographs taken from the Academic Emergency Medicine journal, the official journal of the Society for Academic Emergency Medicine. Topics covered include pediatric penile swelling, right index finger pain, left leg pain and swelling, insect bite to left leg, vaginal bleeding for one day, abdominal pain, painful red eye, scrotal pain, difficulty breathing, bilateral thigh pain. The case studies here are provided on the Web by EMBBS.

http://www.emedicine.com/emerg/

This online textbook from eMedicine (from the Boston Medical Publishing Corp) provides information on a wide range of emergency medicine topics; Emergency Medical Systems; Epidemiology; Implantable Devices; Legal Aspects of Emergency Medicine; Legislation; Managing the Emergency Department; Medical Topics; Organizations in Emergency Medicine; Special Aspects of Emergency Medicine; and Special Aspects of Foreign and Missionary Emergency Medicine. Each chapter is written by physicians, who regularly update their chapter periodically. Each chapter has full author and editor details, with contact e-mail addresses, and how far the chapter has been completed. There is a self test after some of the chapters.

General Medicine

http://www.uptodate.com/

Possibly one of the best sites available for focussed up to date reviews for the non specialist in any given area of general internal medicine: this will last you through to post MRCP and consultant posts. Subscription only.

Appendix

Conclusion

It is important to evaluate critically new sites that you find on the internet. Who is/are the author(s)? What are their qualifications? How often is the review or article updated?

We are convinced that computers and the Internet are a great ally for anyone wanting to pass MRCP part 1 (and eventually part 2). We hope that in addition to the book this article will be an added bonus for those starting out with no prior knowledge of the subject. Good luck!

Callum B Pearce

Ray McCrudden